*Anyone caring for a parent, partner, friend or ¢
discover here a rich, compellingly-written guide
Rothman are wise and gentle mentors.*

—Neil Chethik, syndic
author of *FatherLoss:*
With the Deaths of Th

**DO NOT WRITE IN
WORKBOOKS
Please copy pages or work
on a separate sheet**

I'LL TAKE
CARE OF YOU

A Practical Guide for Family Caregivers

Joseph A. Ilardo, Ph.D., L.C.S.W.
Carole R. Rothman, Ph.D.

New Harbinger Publications, Inc.

Publisher's Note

This publication is designed to provide accurate and authoritative information in regard to the subject matter covered. It is sold with the understanding that the publisher is not engaged in rendering psychological, financial, legal, or other professional services. If expert assistance or counseling is needed, the services of a competent professional should be sought.

Distributed in the U.S.A. by Publishers Group West; in Canada by Raincoast Books; in Great Britain by Airlift Book Company, Ltd.; in South Africa by Real Books, Ltd.; in Australia by Boobook; and in New Zealand by Tandem Press.

Copyright © 1999 by Joseph A. Ilardo and Carole R. Rothman
New Harbinger Publications, Inc.
5674 Shattuck Avenue
Oakland, CA 94609

Cover design by Blue Design
Edited by Kayla Sussell
Text design by Michele Waters

Library of Congress Catalog Card Number: 99-74368
ISBN 1-57224-165-9 Paperback

Printed in the United States of America

New Harbinger Publications' Website address: www.newharbinger.com

01   00

10   9   8   7   6   5   4   3   2

To my mother, the most loving caregiver I have ever known and the most generous recipient imaginable, and to my co-author, Carole Rothman, who has enriched not just this book, but my thinking, my heart, and my life.

Joseph Ilardo

Dedicated to the memory of my grandfather, Benjamin Rabinowitz, who opened my mind, and to my co-author, Joe Ilardo, who opened my heart.

Carole Rothman

Contents

PART II
COPING AS A CAREGIVER

ACKNOWLEDGMENTS

We wish to thank our students, patients, and friends for their help in writing this book, most especially the members of the caregiver support groups we ran, the social workers and other professionals who offered experiences and insights, and the families who shared their stories with us.

Nancy Bialo-Karagis, Psy.D., School Psychologist, and Diane Kissner, M.A., Reading Specialist, Windward School, offered especially insightful comments about special needs children. Hope Knutsson's contributions to the chapter on long-distance caregiving improved it immeasurably.

Kristin Beck and Kayla Sussell at New Harbinger Publications, partners in the process of bringing this book to completion, have been enthusiastic and insightful. Their editorial suggestions and responsiveness have helped shape the book in important ways.

Finally, we wish to thank Jon Rothman for so ably preparing many of his own meals during the writing of this book, and our other children—Dan Rothman, Janine Tesbir, and Karen Ilardo—for their support and interest.

INTRODUCTION

This book is for all caregivers, regardless of the age or special needs of the person for whom they provide care.

"I'll take care of you, Mommy!" said the solemn little boy. He allowed his mother to unzip his coat. "Thank you, honey," she smiled. "Mommy will be fine. I just need to see the doctor so he can give me some medicine for my cold." She was patient and appreciative. The little boy looked directly into her eyes and hesitated a moment. "OK!" he said with relief and tenderness. As he wandered over to the toy station in the waiting room, he looked over his shoulder and said lovingly, "But I will, you know!"

The scene took only seconds, but it said a great deal. "I'll take care of you" captures a spontaneous, loving impulse. It is an expression of caring and devotion. Caregiving is as natural a process as learning to walk. In a sense, we are all caregivers and care recipients. Throughout our lives, we inevitably move in and out of these roles. However, learning how to be a caregiver isn't automatic. And, sometimes, we are thrust into this role without preparation. An auto accident can transform an able-bodied spouse into a care recipient for life. So can a diagnosis of a chronic illness such as multiple sclerosis (MS). The birth of a special needs child can change a couple's future.

Is This Book for You?

This book is intended for all caregivers, regardless of the age or needs of their care recipients.

It is for you if you have aging or elderly parents. You are a caregiver regardless of whether they can manage with minimal help, or whether they require extensive assistance with everyday tasks such as shopping, paying bills, perhaps even eating, dressing, and bathing.

It is for you if you are the parent of a child with a physical, cognitive, or emotional disability. You may not even view yourself as a caregiver, since giving care is an integral part of parenthood. However, your responsibilities go far beyond those usually associated with raising children.

It is for you if you are taking care of a chronically ill or disabled partner or spouse, or any other adult family member. Whenever one individual's responsibilities for the physical or emotional well-being of another require extraordinary time, energy, and effort, that person can be called a caregiver.

This book is for you if you are a "hidden caregiver," providing support, guidance, or protection for a person who is not identified as "ill" or as having "special needs" yet requires consideration or adaptation that goes beyond the norm. Your care recipient may be a dependent spouse, an emotionally needy sibling, or a dysfunctional business associate. As a hidden caregiver, you may spend enormous amounts of time and energy maintaining a workable relationship with this person, while still accomplishing whatever other tasks need to be done. For instance, if your husband is a hidden care recipient, you must not only maintain peace and stability in your marriage, you must also take care of him while running the household, and raising children. Furthermore, you may well find that your children are also burdened with the task of caregiving. They, too, may feel responsible for their father's well-being, serving as his companion at the expense of their own peer relationships.

This book is also for you if you are providing care under circumstances that set you apart from other caregivers. For example, if you have an illness or disability that affects your own functioning, you are, in effect, a caregiver for two. If you are a long-distance caregiver, you must contend with the inconvenience and expense of travel and arrange for necessary coverage in your absence. And, if you cannot get cooperation—from siblings, current family members, or your employer—your caregiving is necessarily affected by this additional burden.

Why This Book Is Unique

This book is unlike similar ones because we address topics that are rarely discussed in books about caregiving. For example, we show how to accept and deal constructively with thoughts, feelings, and fantasies usually considered unthinkable and unacceptable— such as feeling rage toward your care recipient. We discuss the impact of the death of the care recipient, not only when it is expected (e.g., from a terminal illness), but when it is unexpected (e.g., from a suicide). We stress the importance of maintaining realistic expectations as a caregiver. Neither you nor your care recipient is likely to change in temperament when you become a caregiver. If you are laid back, cheerful, and easygoing, you will most likely carry those traits over to your caregiving. If you tend to become anxious easily, or are meticulous and perfectionistic, that will be reflected, as well. If your mother was never gracious and nothing you ever did pleased her, don't expect her to be grateful and uncomplaining now. Just as no amount of effort can give a tiger spots or a leopard stripes, personality traits tend to be well ingrained. By knowing yourself and the person you are caring for, you can recognize trouble spots early, and spare yourself grief.

Another unique feature of this book is its attention to managing emotionally disturbed family members who are part of the caregiving team. A mentally ill sibling or an alcoholic uncle may truly wish to be helpful, yet be unaware that their very presence exacerbates the usual difficulties that caregivers and their recipients face.

Our orientation is practical and helpful. This is reflected in two ways. First, we have avoided burdening you with irrelevant data and references. We have included references only when appropriate and when they are likely to be of use. Second, we have included exercises, activities, and inventories that can help you to better understand yourself and your situation. The more you understand, the more successful you will be in meeting your care recipient's needs. Charts and forms are provided, to help you record information in a useful and organized manner. These should prove invaluable when you must document facts or when you meet with health-care providers, teachers, or other professionals whose cooperation you need.

Most of this material, in addition to appearing in the body of the text, is reproduced in the Appendix, pages 171–202. We have done this for two reasons. First, if you would rather not write in the book itself, you can photocopy the activities you need. Second, if you wish to use these for a support group, you can make a copy for each member. For ease of duplication, each activity starts on a separate page.

The activities in the Appendix can also serve as starting points for discussion in caregiver support groups. A special section provides instructions to support group facilitators on how to adapt these activities. Chapter 12 on caregiver support groups and our suggestions for using the exercises in such groups are offered in response to the growth of these groups. This is the only book of its kind to respond directly to this growing need.

A Note on Style

Since caregivers can be male or female, we use the gender-neutral term "caregiver" whenever possible. When it is not possible, we refer to the caregiver as "she" because more than 80 percent of family caregivers are female. However, many men are devoted caregivers, and this book is for them, too.

How to Use This Book

There is great value in understanding the many aspects of caregiving—from the roles of caregiver and care recipient, to avoiding burnout and coping with "unacceptable" feelings. We suggest that you read through the entire book. Nevertheless, each chapter can stand on its own. If you are pressed for time, go directly to the chapters that have relevance to your situation. Use the comprehensive index and the Resources section on pages 203–210 to locate information quickly.

PART ONE

UNDERSTANDING YOUR CAREGIVER ROLE

What does it mean to be a caregiver? If you have taken on this role, either by choice or by circumstance, you are most likely coping with major changes in your own life. The first three chapters of this book focus on you and your care recipient—who you are as individuals, your feelings about this special relationship, the difficulties you are likely to be experiencing—and suggest ways to deal with the emotional and practical issues that arise when one person becomes responsible for the welfare of another.

CHAPTER ONE

BEING A CAREGIVER

In this chapter we define the term caregiver. You will learn how closely you fit the profile of the typical caregiver with regard to the kinds of services you provide, the pressures you are under, and how you happened to become a caregiver. At the end of the chapter, you will be given the opportunity to use your newfound knowledge to plan for any desired changes.

Your Caregiver Profile

A caregiver is an individual who provides care for another person who, ordinarily, would not require care. For example, someone may become a caregiver when a spouse or partner suffers an injury or becomes chronically ill. Similarly, parents are usually responsible for the care of their children, but as parents age, their children become their caregivers. In some cases, the label is applied when the care needed goes far beyond what would normally be required, as when a twelve-year-old brain-damaged child needs to be fed, toileted, and bathed.

Caregiving is actually a two-part process, in which the caregiver first must recognize the needs of the care recipient, then figure out how to meet them. Depending on the nature of the problem, helping may require a small amount of work or a great deal. In the latter case, everyday tasks such as bathing or eating can become tedious chores that take extended periods of time to accomplish.

No matter what tasks they perform, caregivers must be sensitive to their care recipients' feelings about being dependent. When some people need help, they accept it graciously and are cooperative. Others, however, may be difficult, angry, or rude. Disgusted with themselves, furious with life, and enraged at their illness or disability, members of this second group may curse and berate the very people who provide the help they need. Care recipients may be whiny and manipulative or stubborn and resistant. Some become possessive and demanding, resentful of any attempts their caregivers make to take time for themselves. If you are a caregiver and wish to remain sane and helpful, you must not only be a planner, innovator, organizer, and helpmate, but a psychologist as well! You must be accepting, forgiving, understanding, and patient. And, while doing all this, you must attend to your own needs, or you run the risk of burnout. Make no mistake about it, caregiving is anything but easy.

Reactions to Being a Caregiver

Although it is impossible to predict with certainty how a person will react to becoming a caregiver, the following variables help determine the ease with which this role can be assumed. In assessing your own reactions, consider each of the following factors.

The Suddenness with Which You Are Thrust into the Role

Did you expect to become a caregiver? If you are thrown into that role without warning or the chance to prepare emotionally, you may have an unusually difficult time. On the other hand, if you take on that role gradually, adjustment is often easier. This was what happened in the L family. Over many years, Mrs. L, who was healthier than her husband, gradually assumed more and more tasks in caring for him. Toward the end of his life, she almost literally became his eyes and ears. A woman of strong will and boundless energy, she managed to provide most of the care he required until she was in her mid-eighties. A home health aide was brought in (and willingly accepted) only when the limits of the elderly woman's strength and endurance made caregiving impossible. The fact that her responsibilities grew incrementally over the years gave her time to adjust emotionally to the role and to develop needed skills. Not all caregivers have that luxury.

The Phase of Your Life Cycle

As partners age, they expect to provide caregiving services for one another. Health problems and minor surgeries become more common, knees wear out, chronic conditions such as arthritis and high blood pressure take their toll. It is quite another matter when a young person must care for an equally young spouse. For example, a thirty-three-year-old woman, with two small children and a career of her own, had to care for her thirty-five-year-old husband when he was diagnosed with inoperable bone cancer. So many demands fell on this young woman's shoulders at the same time that she was almost crushed beneath their weight. "Everything I counted on was falling apart. How could I face losing my husband? What about the children? My career? His parents? My parents?"

There is never a right time to become the caregiver for a chronically ill or disabled person, but some times are worse than others. For example, the early phases of a family's life cycle are typically characterized by the presence of young children and unsettled finances. If the family has relocated recently (not unusual for young couples), they may also have limited knowledge of the new community and its resources. These factors, when added to caregiving responsibilities, may create more stress than they can handle.

The Anticipated Outcome

Short-term caregiving is much easier to accept because the disability is temporary and the anticipated outcome is a happy one. For example, when one partner cares for another following a surgical procedure from which complete recovery is expected, caregiving is usually short-term and upbeat. Taking on the role of caregiver is far more upsetting and terrifying when there can be no happy ending.

The Quality of the Relationship

The presence of love and mutual respect between partners in their normal interactions increases the likelihood of a generous give-and-take in adverse circumstances. By contrast, when genuine caring is absent, a partner's needs may quickly become burdensome. Caregiving is like a litmus test of the health of the relationship. "Our marriage was always a sham," a woman said recently, in the course of discussing her angry reactions to caring for her husband following a serious accident. "I can't stand taking care of Pete. I knew things weren't good, but I didn't realize they were this bad. I guess I just didn't want to face how little we really have between us."

Sometimes, even prior to the onset of formal caregiving, there is a long history of dependency on the part of one spouse. If the dependent partner becomes ill or disabled, his spouse, worn down by everyday, unacknowledged caregiving, may become resentful of the additional burden. In one instance, following a needy spouse's back surgery, his always-patient wife became contemptuous of her husband's disability and she provided care only grudgingly. (See chapter 7 for more on this subject.)

The Demands on the Caregiver

Some care recipients need care that is easy to deliver. The caregiver's responsibilities may be limited to providing companionship, reminding a partner to take a pill, and driving him/her to the doctor. On the other hand, care recipients may be completely unable to care for themselves, requiring assistance with walking, showering, and even using the toilet.

One elderly couple brought this point home clearly. They were referred for counseling by a neurologist following a worsening of the husband's symptoms of dementia. The problem for which they were referred, however, was his healthy wife's distress. She was nearly overwhelmed by her husband's illness, and made it quite clear that it was she, not he, who needed support. "I don't know if I can cope any longer," she stated sadly. "How can I take care of him when he can't even remember who I am!"

The Care Recipient's Attitude

Care recipients are often far from cooperative. They may be so angry at being ill or disabled that they cannot acknowledge the help they're receiving, let alone express gratitude for it. Feeling sorry for themselves, consumed by self-pity, they cannot appreciate the efforts made on their behalf.

Ironically, however, gratitude and cooperation don't always make things easier. They may have the opposite effect, inhibiting any feelings of anger and resentment the caregiver may have, thereby making her job even more difficult. (See chapter 3 for a more complete discussion of this subject.)

The Caregiver's Temperament

Relaxed, confident, and flexible caregivers are able to assume their burdens with quiet calm, inspiring faith in their care recipients. Conversely, anxious and uncertain caregivers, often edgy themselves, do anything but inspire confidence. Caregivers who know and respect their limitations, and who are willing to ask for help, almost always succeed with less angst than those who feel they must do it all and are unwilling to ask for or accept assistance.

At this point, we would like you to take a few moments to answer some questions about yourself as a caregiver. Throughout this book, we will ask you to respond to questions like these. Your answers may be used as a starting point for discussion in a caregiver support group or to help you identify problems or plan for changes on your own. To derive full benefit from your reading, we ask that you take the time to answer these questions thoughtfully and honestly, and use them as an opportunity to clarify your feelings and needs.

Your Caregiver Profile

Please answer each of the following questions by checking the appropriate box.

1. Your sex:
   - ☐ M
   - ☐ F

2. Your age:
   - ☐ Under 30
   - ☐ 30–39
   - ☐ 40–49
   - ☐ 50–59
   - ☐ 60 or above

3. Your relationships:
   - ☐ Married or live with partner
   - ☐ Single, divorced, separated, or widowed

4. Your responsibilities in addition to caregiving:
   - ☐ Work inside the home
   - ☐ homemaking

- ❑ home-based business
- ❑ care for children under age 18
- ❑ care for children over age 18
- ❑ Work outside the home
  - ❑ parttime employment
  - ❑ fulltime employment

5. Percent of caregiving responsibilities that fall on you:

- ❑ 100% (you are the sole caregiver)
- ❑ You share caregiving responsibilities with others
  - ❑ bulk (more than 50%) of caregiving responsibilities fall on you
  - ❑ bulk of caregiving responsibilities fall on one or more other persons

6. The person for whom you provide care:

- ❑ spouse or partner
- ❑ child
- ❑ parent
- ❑ sibling, friend, relative, or other

Compare your answers to those of the typical caregiver. The following data, collected and reported by both the National Family Caregivers Association (National Family Caregivers Association 1998), indicate that the typical family caregiver is female (82%), married (74%), and between thirty-six and sixty-five years old. She is likely to be employed (47%) and to work more than thirty-one hours a week (71%).

Most caregivers care for a spouse or partner (48%). A smaller percentage cares for a parent (24%). Nineteen percent provide care for children; the remainder (9%) care for a sibling, friend, relative, or some other person.

The typical female family caregiver often gets little help. When the care recipients are elderly parents, male siblings are likely to provide moral support and sometimes financial help, but little more. Female siblings sometimes cooperate, although one daughter often assumes the bulk of the responsibility. For example, in one case a dutiful daughter cared for both of her elderly parents while her less responsible sister remained uninvolved, doing little more than calling her parents occasionally and visiting them once in a great while. Sadly, on the few occasions when she and her sister did make time to discuss the disparity in their responsibilities, the uninvolved sibling almost always called her sister a martyr and a fool.

Caregiver Pressures

Family caregivers experience many different pressures. Some can be traced to external factors. Others originate within the caregivers themselves.

Typical External Pressures

Your spouse complains that you are unavailable. He may say that "Even when you're here physically, you're not here emotionally." Your children resent the fact that you're always so busy you have no time for them. Your boss and colleagues tolerate your personal phone calls, occasional absences, late arrivals, and early departures. However, tolerant as they may be, they make it known that they still expect you will fulfill your job responsibilities. Your siblings simply expect that you will be able to do it all. Your friends become impatient with you because you cancel social engagements, fail to return calls, and drop out of touch for long periods of time. In each of these instances, you feel pressure. Whether subtle or direct, it is burdensome.

Unusual External Pressures

Often caregivers must cope with additional stress unrelated to caregiving. Some may be under extreme financial pressure. Others are facing divorce. Still others may have just lost a job. These additional stressors put the caregiver at risk for overload and burnout, and demand special vigilance with regard to self-care. The coping strategies discussed below will be especially useful for caregivers in these potentially explosive situations.

Internal Pressures

In addition to pressures that originate externally, caregivers sometimes impose pressures on themselves. For instance, you may expect that regardless of the number and kinds of responsibilities you must fulfill, you should be able to carry them off without letting anyone down. One woman berated herself for her inability to take care of her ill husband while simultaneously looking after her three children, running a business, and caring for her own elderly parents. Only after she thought about her predicament did she come to realize that she simply could not do all she wished. Other pressures are the result of loneliness and isolation. Friends may drift away because they have never lived through your situation and cannot appreciate the trials you are experiencing.

As a caregiver, you probably live with almost constant feelings of frustration. Coping with a loved one's temporary disability is difficult enough. When age, permanent disability, long-term health problems, a chronic mental disorder, or a terminal illness makes any prospect of recovery impossible, the situation is indeed depressing.

Leisure time is a phrase that may well have lost meaning for you. You are not alone. Many caregivers complain of a lack of leisure and personal time.

The Caregiving Services You Provide

There are different kinds and degrees of caregiving responsibilities. Some caregivers are little more than companions to their care recipients. They may read to their care recipients or bring them lunch. These are relatively simple services—neither physically taxing nor emotionally demanding. On the other hand, the caregiver may become the eyes, ears, and mind of the recipient.

Often, caregiving responsibilities change over time. For example, when you provide care for an aging individual, it's typical for demands to increase as time passes. To gauge the kind of caregiving responsibilities you have, please complete the following questionnaire:

Caregiving Services

Please put a checkmark on the appropriate lines.

1. As a caregiver, I primarily:

　　____ Provide companionship and show concern through calls and occasional visits

　　____ Take my care recipient to lunch

____ Shop with my care recipient

____ Arrange for occasional outings

2. As a caregiver, I primarily:

____ Arrange medical appointments, coordinate schedules, etc.

____ Take my care recipient to medical appointments; provide transport for laboratory tests, and take him/her to and from procedures (such as surgeries) performed on an outpatient basis

____ Consult with members of my care recipient's health-care team and make decisions in consultation with my care recipient

____ Shop for my care recipient

____ Prepare some meals for my care recipient

3. As a caregiver, I primarily:

____ Provide homemaking services (do laundry, clean house, etc.)

____ Arrange for home repairs, maintenance, etc.

____ Prepare most or all meals

____ Arrange for care when I can't be there

____ Pay bills

4. As a caregiver, I primarily:

____ Provide help with bathing, dressing, eating, and using the toilet

____ Assist with the management of incontinence

____ Help my care recipient cope despite serious cognitive disabilities (for example, the forgetfulness and lack of orientation characteristic of Alzheimer's disease)

____ Arrange for home-health aides and others to provide help when I am not available

5. As a caregiver, I primarily:

____ Help my care recipient prepare advance directives such as a living will

____ Serve as health care proxy

____ Serve as attorney-in-fact for most or all other matters; manage all financial affairs, etc.

The items in this questionnaire were arranged in five clusters of caregiving activities. Each cluster represents a different degree of responsibility. See the table below:

Cluster Number	Description
1.	Light duty (companionship, socialization)
2.	Medium duty (oversight, transport, consultation, and practical assistance)
3.	Substantial duty
4.	Heavy duty (services essential for living)
5.	Legal, ethical, and moral responsibilities

Items in the higher number or later clusters are usually added to those in the lower number or earlier clusters, rather than simply replacing them. For example, providing companionship does not end when medical oversight and transport are added to your caregiving responsibilities. As time passes, and as a care recipient ages or becomes sicker, the caregiver takes on more and more responsibilities. Little wonder that the death of a recipient sometimes evokes not only sadness, but relief and anxiety as well. "What will I do now?" is a question more than one caregiver has asked herself when her care recipient has died.

How You Became a Caregiver

Why do certain family members become caregivers while others do not? Under what conditions does an individual take on this role? Is the decision made because of social expectations? Gender? The relationship with the care recipient? Accident or circumstances? Family pressures? Timing? Physical proximity to the person(s) needing care? Consider the following examples:

1. Several years after Rosemary married Carl, he was stricken with myasthenia gravis, a chronic and debilitating condition. Since she was his wife, it seemed most reasonable that she would assume responsibility for his care.

2. When Dr. and Mrs. Shapiro's third child was born with a serious brain disease, it seemed natural that they would serve as her caregivers.

3. When, by second grade, it became clear that Brian was learning disabled, his mother assumed responsibility for advocating

on his behalf, attending parent-teacher conferences, and ensuring that he got the extra help he required. Because his father worked outside the home in a job that required frequent travel, his mother, Sharon, seemed the logical person to assume responsibility for his care.

4. As Jose's parents grew older and became infirm, it seemed logical that Jose and his wife would be the ones to care for them; Jose's brother, Manuel, had never been very close to either of his parents. Furthermore, Jose had long been the "good" child in the family.

5. Tahitia had always been considered the "crazy" one in her family: sensitive, deeply feeling, and intelligent, she had never really been understood by her parents or her younger sister, Mavis. Although their father died when the girls were in their late twenties, their mother lived on for many years. Mavis automatically assumed responsibility for her care. The fact that this placed all the responsibility on her shoulders was considered an acceptable price to pay for maintaining peace in the family.

6. When Mrs. Borruso, eighty-one, began showing signs of dementia, her husband, Emil, eighty-three, assumed the role of caregiver. However, despite his good intentions, he was not really up to the task. This placed their daughter in a predicament. Whenever she attempted to intervene, Mr. Borruso rebuffed her efforts. "I had to pretend my father was taking care of Mom," she observed, "while, in fact, the responsibility fell on me."

As these examples illustrate, many circumstances contribute to a person becoming a caregiver. The key factors are: social expectations, relationship quality, self-perceptions, and accident and circumstances. Often, two or more factors combine to determine the decision.

Social Expectations

In most societies, ours included, there are unwritten expectations about who will care for whom in the event that caregiving becomes necessary. For example, if a child is ill, disabled, or born with a birth defect, it is *expected* that the parents will assume responsibility if at all possible. If a spouse or domestic partner becomes ill or is injured, it is assumed that the able-bodied partner will become the caregiver. Similarly, as a person ages, it is the life partner who usually provides care until that is no longer possible. At that point their children, if there are any, will take on the job of providing care. Institutionalization is socially sanctioned only when the situation becomes unmanageable, and even then, it is often accompanied by recriminations and guilt.

Within the realm of social expectations, gender becomes a factor. In most societies, women are expected to be caregivers as a natural extension of their nurturing role. Although men can be wonderfully compassionate, they are not commonly expected to take on this responsibility.

Convenience is also a factor. It is usually assumed that the person who lives closest to the care recipient and whose schedule is the most flexible will become the caregiver. This may, unfortunately, result in a resentful caregiver who feels boxed in and unable to refuse the role because it makes "so much sense" for her to take it on.

To provide a sense of the rules that govern decisions about who assumes caregiving responsibilities, we have created a decision tree that reflects what we have observed. Our goal is not to include every conceivable situation in which care is required, only the most common ones.

Two other family-related variables play a role. The first one is past behaviors within the family. In every family, some members are simply more solicitous, more accommodating, and more willing to put themselves out for others. If a person has earned that reputation, it's likely he or she will become a caregiver when the need arises.

The second variable is birth order. For one thing, age is often tied to status in families, even among adult children. For that reason, younger adult children, perhaps the youngest, will be charged with caregiving responsibilities. For another, the youngest adult child may still be living at home when the need for caregiving arises and the older siblings may have been on their own for some time.

Relationship Quality

All other things being equal, the person who has the closest and most gratifying relationship with the care recipient is most likely to become the caregiver. Often this is the favorite child. This was the case in the O'Brien family. Margaret was the apple of her parents' eye. Her sister, by contrast, had always been a source of distress. Rebellious and self-absorbed, Nora had provided little gratification to her hard-working parents. It was thus logical that when it came time to provide care, Margaret would take on those responsibilities.

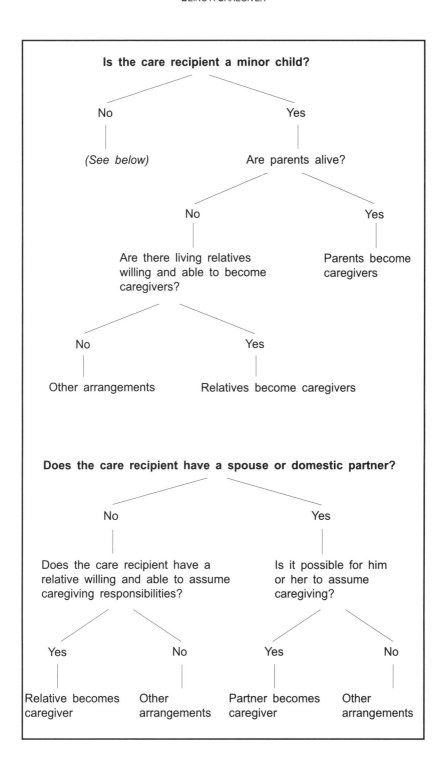

Is the care recipient a minor child?

No — *(See below)*

Yes — Are parents alive?

No — Are there living relatives willing and able to become caregivers?

Yes — Parents become caregivers

No — Other arrangements

Yes — Relatives become caregivers

Does the care recipient have a spouse or domestic partner?

No — Does the care recipient have a relative willing and able to assume caregiving responsibilities?

Yes — Is it possible for him or her to assume caregiving?

Yes — Relative becomes caregiver

No — Other arrangements

Yes — Partner becomes caregiver

No — Other arrangements

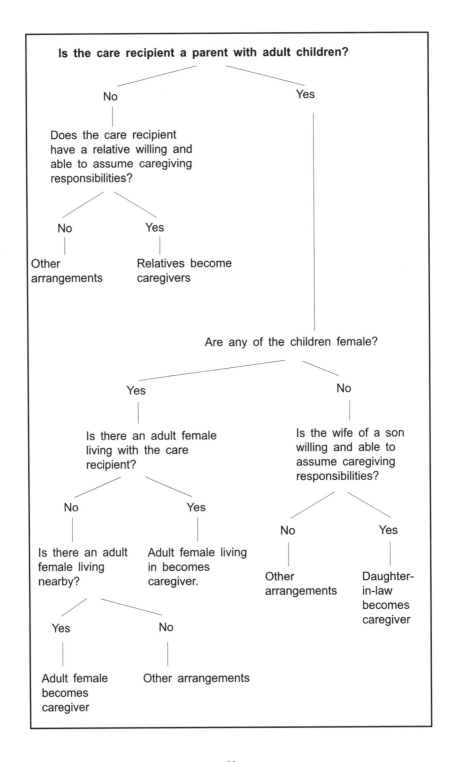

Self-Perception

Self-perception almost always plays a part in determining the choice of caregiver. If a person sees herself as caring, devoted, reliable, and so on, she will likely assume the role. Since terms such as caring, kind, and compassionate are more often applied to women than men, it's not surprising that women are assigned the caregiving role, and that they are also most likely to see themselves as fitting the part perfectly.

It's also likely that a good many caregivers assume that role because it suits them temperamentally. Something in their personality makes them capable of tolerating the demands of caregiving. Indeed, some caregivers take genuine pleasure in their work. Here, for example, is the response of a caregiver who attended one of our workshops. When asked about the rewards of caregiving, she wrote: "I think my caregiving has made me a better person." These are some of the benefits:

1. A new relationship with person being cared for (in her case, it was an elderly mother)
2. A chance to give back
3. A sense of accomplishment
4. Development of new skills, knowledge (e.g., advocacy abilities)
5. Increased compassion and personal growth
6. New relationships with others through support groups
7. The building of memories

Sometimes, however, the motives underlying an apparent desire to provide care are not at all benign. Some caregivers, for example, take perverse pleasure in playing the martyr, simultaneously "upstaging" other family members and inducing guilt. "See what a good child I am," they say by their self-sacrifice. Others do it for more sinister reasons, such as to take financial advantage of the care recipient. It would be unfair to defame all caregivers by assuming they are driven by unhealthy motives. Yet it would be naive to assume that love and compassion are the only motives involved.

Accident and Circumstances

Some people are thrust into the role of caregiver by accident and circumstances. As the table above suggests, if one's child requires special care, it falls on the parent to assume the job.

Similarly, if one's partner is disabled or stricken with an illness, it is the other's responsibility to see the loved one through the ordeal. Likewise, an only child, or the only caring one, usually takes care of aging parents.

Such caregivers may not delight in what they must do. They may actually hate it, but they believe that they have little choice. Under such circumstances, it is healthier to face the anger and resentment at having been forced to assume the role than to suppress such feelings. (See chapter 3.)

The checklist on the following pages is intended to heighten your awareness of how you happened to become a caregiver. After you have completed it, you will have a chance to review your results, identify any changes you wish to make, and formulate an appropriate action plan.

Why You Became a Caregiver

Instructions: Please indicate the extent to which, in your opinion, each factor resulted in your becoming a caregiver. Mark each scale at the appropriate point.

1. **Social Expectations**

    I have become a caregiver because of

    a. my sex

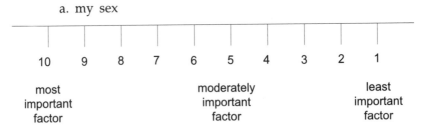

    b. family pressures: my role and past experiences in my family made me the most likely choice

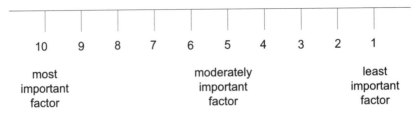

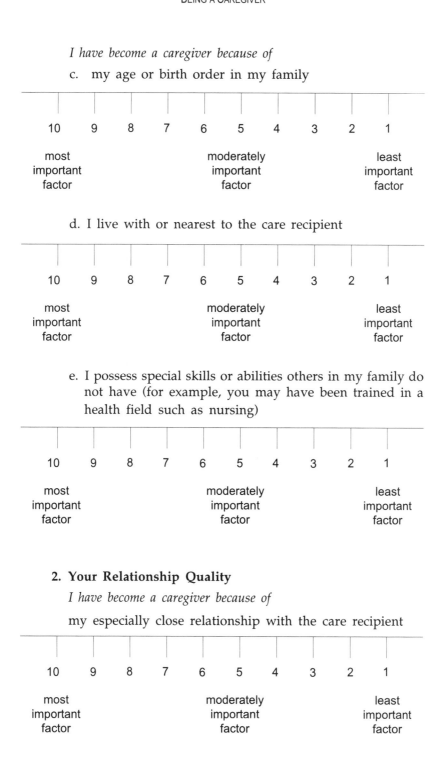

I have become a caregiver because of

c. my age or birth order in my family

| 10 | 9 | 8 | 7 | 6 | 5 | 4 | 3 | 2 | 1 |

most important factor | moderately important factor | least important factor

d. I live with or nearest to the care recipient

| 10 | 9 | 8 | 7 | 6 | 5 | 4 | 3 | 2 | 1 |

most important factor | moderately important factor | least important factor

e. I possess special skills or abilities others in my family do not have (for example, you may have been trained in a health field such as nursing)

| 10 | 9 | 8 | 7 | 6 | 5 | 4 | 3 | 2 | 1 |

most important factor | moderately important factor | least important factor

2. Your Relationship Quality

I have become a caregiver because of

my especially close relationship with the care recipient

| 10 | 9 | 8 | 7 | 6 | 5 | 4 | 3 | 2 | 1 |

most important factor | moderately important factor | least important factor

3. Self-Perceptions

I have become a caregiver because

a. I see myself as strong, reliable, and competent

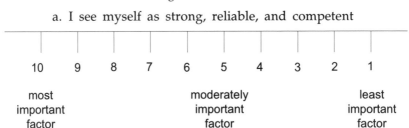

10	9	8	7	6	5	4	3	2	1

most important factor   moderately important factor   least important factor

b. I am nurturing and enjoy caring for others

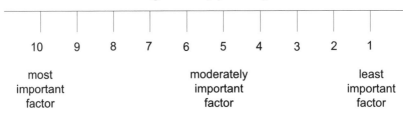

10	9	8	7	6	5	4	3	2	1

most important factor   moderately important factor   least important factor

c. I enjoy being needed, and take pleasure in being seen as the grateful child or the devoted parent

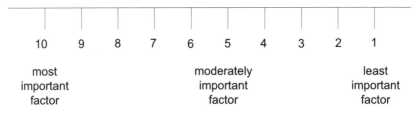

10	9	8	7	6	5	4	3	2	1

most important factor   moderately important factor   least important factor

d. I am willing to defer satisfaction of my own needs to help others

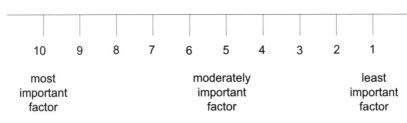

10	9	8	7	6	5	4	3	2	1

most important factor   moderately important factor   least important factor

4. Accident and Circumstances

I have become a caregiver because of

illness, accident, or other circumstances beyond my control

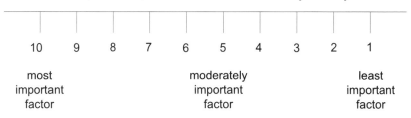

10	9	8	7

| 10 | 9 | 8 | 7 | 6 | 5 | 4 | 3 | 2 | 1 |

most
important
factor

moderately
important
factor

least
important
factor

By plotting your scores on each criterion in the box on page 26, you can get a sense of the factors that contributed to your assuming the caregiving role. If your examination of the results of this inventory suggests that you need or want to re-evaluate your position, this is the time to begin thinking about that.

Instructions: Each item in Column A corresponds to each question you just completed. In Column B, record the numeric score you marked above. Then plot the numbers on the grid that appears at the bottom of this exercise.

Column A

Factor

Column B

Score You Earned
(10 = most important,
1 = least)

1. Social Expectations

Sex _____

Family pressures: roles and past
experiences in the family _____

Age or birth order _____

Physical proximity to care recipient _____

Special skills and abilities _____

2. Relationship Quality (emotional
closeness to care recipient) _____

3. Self-Perceptions

See myself as strong, reliable, and
competent _____

Nurturing personality _____

Enjoy being needed _____

Willing to defer personal satisfaction

_____

4. Accident and Circumstances _____

Now plot on the grid below the number score you wrote on each
line:

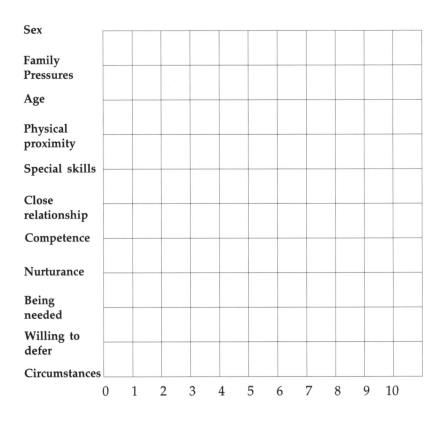

Plan of Action

Take a moment now to review your questionnaire results. If you are comfortable with the factors responsible for your becoming a caregiver, and do not resent having taken on this role, then go no further. If, however, this is not true of you, use the Action Plan Example below to plan for some changes. For example, if you care for your mother because you live on the next block, find a way to involve your brother, who lives elsewhere. If you were chosen as caregiver because you are the only "girl" in the family, or the youngest child, address this issue with your siblings and arrange for a more equitable distribution of responsibilities.

In the following box, we have included an example of an Action Plan. It consists of a goal, the means to achieve it, and measures to evaluate outcomes. Use it as a guide for your own planning.

Action Plan Example

1. Things I'd Like to Change (my goal): I need assistance in taking care of my mother.
2. Methods (how I can achieve my goal)
   a. I can call my siblings, spell out what I am doing for Mom, and ask them to help out.
   b. I can call a home health agency and arrange for an aide to come twice a week.
   c. I can arrange for meals-on-wheels so I don't have to cook for Mom as often.
3. Measure(s) of Success (how I will know I have accomplished what I set out to do):
   a. I will have more time for myself and my family.
   b. I will feel better about taking care of Mom.
   c. I'll be less resentful and less tired.

CHAPTER TWO

THE DYNAMICS OF CAREGIVING

In this chapter, we offer practical suggestions to help you cope with the changes that occur when people take on the interdependent roles of caregiver and care recipient. We look closely at the dynamics involved, at how the relationship is redefined, and at issues of dependency and control.

When Jennifer received word that her husband had been injured on the job, she thought little of it. Ted had worked in construction for almost ten years and he had had his share of accidents and injuries. She assumed he'd be laid up for a while, as he had been many times before, then resume life as usual. They'd even come to cherish the last few periods of recovery, since it gave them a chance to be close, and the boys to spend more time with their father. And, to make up for the money they'd lose, she could increase her hours at work.

"Daddy'll be fine," she assured her two sons, who had overheard the phone conversation. "I'll be back from the hospital in a little while, and I'll give you all the details!" Her voice was confident. She breezed through the house gathering keys, jacket, and a snack for Ted. (From the time they met, he had always been partial to Hershey's with almonds.) A slight edge of anxiety gripped her on the way to the hospital. She hadn't liked the serious tone of the nurse who called. "What if . . .?" she began thinking. Then she caught herself, reached for the radio, and tuned to her favorite music station. "Don't start, Jen!" she admonished herself, knowing the ease with which she could begin worrying. "Don't do this to yourself."

When she arrived at the hospital, as she watched the automatic door slide open before her, she heard the sounds of voices, the distant ring of a telephone, and the tinny, singsong voice on the loudspeaker: "Dr. Cahn, please call extension two-seven. Dr. Barry Cahn . . ." Then she entered the white, dizzying world of the emergency room waiting area.

"Jennifer Frith," she said, managing a smile, when the receptionist greeted her brightly from her seat behind the low counter. "My husband, Ted, was brought in a little while ago." There was a pause as the receptionist looked through her records. The woman appeared to be young. Probably new. She took her time. "Ted Frith," she mused aloud. "Yes! Oh, yes!" She seemed satisfied with herself. She read the note, then looked up and met Jennifer's eyes. "He's been taken in to surgery, Mrs. Frith." She smiled, quite inappropriately and rather stupidly, Jennifer thought. "You need to go to the third floor and ask for Dr. Shaffer. He's the doctor overseeing . . ."

"Surgery?" Jennifer interrupted. "What surgery?" Her voice had an edge.

"I don't have any more information," the receptionist interrupted politely. "I just came on shift. You need to go to the third floor." She pointed. "The elevator is just outside that door on the left." The comment was a dismissal. Jennifer turned, murmured a thank-you, and reminded herself to stay calm.

Much of the rest of the afternoon is lost to her now. She remembers walking to the elevator, pressing the small black button with the little white arrow that was almost worn away. She remembers waiting in the corridor as other hospital visitors gathered to await the elevator. She has no recollection of arriving at the third floor. She cannot recall how she had found Dr. Shaffer, and has no clear memory of him. Over the next few months, he became one of a dozen names she saw on hospital bills and wrote countless times on insurance forms.

"Left leg," she remembers someone saying. "Crushed when the backhoe overturned. . . ." She recalls no other words, just the tightening in her gut that has not left her since that afternoon at the hospital. She has a partial recollection of someone who had looked familiar. The woman had been kind, inviting her to sit in an office as she regained her composure. She remembers crying, seeing the Hershey bar fall to the floor while she fumbled in her purse for her handkerchief.

Jennifer's life changed permanently that day. Ted was never able to return to work. The amputation had been unavoidable. And even when the prosthesis was fitted many months after the accident, they never said anything to each other about his job. They knew without discussing it that talking about the accident and his loss would have been too painful for either of them to bear.

Rehabilitation specialists, physical therapists, occupational therapists, orthopedists, neurologists—a cadre of health-care professionals entered their lives. There were endless appointments, countless trips to the hospital and rehabilitation centers. At first, the pain was the most difficult part of their new lives. Neither of them could understand how Ted's left leg could hurt so much when it wasn't there. ("It's called 'phantom limb pain,'" Dr. Fiore explained.)

Over many months, they both came to realize that nothing would ever again return to normal. They had run the entire gamut of human emotions. They had cried together. They had put up a brave front for their sons, Alan and Richard. They'd accepted the kindness of friends. They had even arranged a family outing to a theme park.

But serious changes had taken place in their relationship. Ted, usually even-tempered, had begun showing signs of impatience. Frustrated and in pain, he had "lost it" more than once, raging at the boys for doing nothing more than squabbling as pre-teens always do. Jennifer had come to their defense, a little resentful that so much at home was revolving around Ted's moods. She felt herself becoming something other than a wife to Ted—something more like a mother or a nurse. And Ted, usually strong and definite, had become more like a child—a disagreeable man-child, with the disposition of a demanding and petulant teenager. He gained weight, and she nagged him about it. "What do you want from me, Jen?" he asked angrily. "I can't do much. But I can still eat!" he said bitterly. And even though she tried very hard to avoid admitting it to herself, she found his self-pity disgusting.

Jennifer and Ted never stopped being wife and husband. However, their relationship and the implicit contract that existed between them underwent profound changes. For their marriage to survive, they would have to acknowledge their new reality and find ways to cope with it.

In the following section we discuss the nature of the contract that exists between you and your care recipient. Then we describe how to use your contract to clarify and strengthen your caregiving relationship.

Defining the Relationship

Think of a satisfying relationship you have with someone close to you—a spouse or partner, a sibling, or a good friend. Picture the person in your mind's eye, and conjure up the good feelings you share. Why do things click between the two of you? What do you agree about? Do you share expectations about the relationship? What is likely to happen between the two of you, and what isn't?

Now we'll ask you to do something that may sound a bit odd. We would like you to think about this relationship as a contractual one. A contract, as you know, is an agreement between two people—landlord and tenant, employer and employee, lender and borrower. Every contract spells out rights and responsibilities. It makes clear what each party is expected to do and what each has a right to receive in return. For example, tenants who lease an apartment from a landlord are expected to pay the rent. In return they have the right to the "quiet enjoyment" of the apartment. In his classic work, *The Presentation of Self in Everyday Life* (1959), Erving Goffman extends this concept of contracts to relationships. Here's an example:

When Sherry was seventeen, she was dating a number of young men. Among her male friends, there was one fellow she did not date. Bill was a chum or a pal to her. She could talk to him about anything, including the other guys, confident that he would listen, take her concerns seriously, and offer honest feedback. He was not a boyfriend in the usual sense—just a very good friend who happened to be male.

One day, Sherry and Bill decided to go to a movie. As they sat in the dark theater watching a tender love story, Sherry became aware that Bill had placed his arm around the back of her seat. His hand had crept to her shoulder, and he was gently pulling her toward him. "I felt so weird at that moment!" she said. "It was like incest or something! Here was this guy—my friend!—and he was making a move on me!"

She turned to look at Bill. He was smiling a little timidly, not knowing how Sherry would react. When she pulled away and gently removed his hand from her shoulder, he was crestfallen. They both returned their attention to the movie, but neither watched much of it. The moment had been upsetting to both of them.

Bill and Sherry's experience illustrates the fact that every relationship is governed by a contract, containing terms to which both parties agree. In this case, the relationship between Sherry and Bill had been defined as a close, but platonic, friendship. Romantic or sexual feelings were not to be a part of it. When Bill pulled her to him, he was in effect proposing that they redefine their relationship. He had begun to fall in love with her. Once he had "made his move," Sherry had only two options: She could accept the proposed redefinition, snuggle up to him, and invite further intimacy. Or she could do what she did.

Now, think back to the satisfying relationship we asked you to think about at the start of this section. Use the space below to identify expectations, rights, and responsibilities. First, write down one or two things you expect from your relationship partner.

Second, list a few of his or her expectations of you. Next, identify two or three rights you have in the relationship—things you can do that will be accepted as normal by your partner. Next, identify your partner's rights. Finally, identify your responsibilities and those of your partner—the obligations you each assume by virtue of your involvement with each other.

Terms of Informal Interpersonal Contracts

Expectations

1. Things I expect of my relationship partner (for example, you might expect a good friend to remember your birthday, your sibling to feed your cats when you go away, or your spouse to schedule vacations to coincide with your time off work).

_____

_____

_____

2. Things my relationship partner expects of me (for example, a good friend might expect you to remember her birthday, a younger sibling might expect you to help with homework, and your spouse might expect you to take out the garbage).

_____

_____

_____

Rights

1. My rights (for example, you have the right to get off the phone with your friend if you don't feel like talking any longer).

_____

_____

_____

2. My relationship partner's rights (for example, your sibling may have the right to ask you to lower the volume on your CD player).

_____

_____

_____

Responsibilities

1. My responsibilities (for example, you might feel obligated to do your share around the house).

_____

_____

_____

2. My relationship partner's responsibilities (for example, your spouse may be in charge of changing the oil in the family car).

_____

_____

_____

Now, suppose that you became a caregiver to the person you've been thinking about. Imagine that he or she were seriously disabled in an accident. What would change? Your expectations? Your rights? Your responsibilities? Those of your relationship partner? Take it even further and ask yourself what changes would take place in the satisfactions you both enjoy? The future you envision?

It should not take more than a moment to realize that when one person becomes a caregiver to another, the definition of the relationship changes profoundly. In the case of Jennifer and Ted, everything changed.

Dependency and Control

The delicate and sensitive issues of dependency and control arise whenever one person becomes responsible for another. The care recipient is, of necessity, dependent on the caregiver, and may have strong feelings about this. The caregiver's task is to assume responsibility, but not at the expense of the recipient's dignity. And so, the question arises: How can these issues be resolved?

At first it may seem strange to pose such a question. After all, the caregiver is obviously in control, isn't she? It's she who is ablebodied, and makes many of the decisions. The care recipient, on the other hand, is the person in need. He relies on the caregiver to provide the services he requires. Although it seems unlikely that a person in such a dependent position could be in control of the relationship, he can.

Sometimes one person's reliance on another enables the dependent person to dictate what happens in the relationship. For example, a woman who is afraid to drive on highways makes it necessary for her husband to drive her when she needs to go somewhere. Similarly, a husband who assumes the role of "domestic incompetent" and relies on his wife to perform even the simplest household tasks, can keep her captive in a subtle way. In such situations the "strong" and "able" partner is responding to the implicit demands of the person in need.

Care Recipient Control

You may not realize that your care recipient is controlling you. To discover whether he is, pay attention to the timing of his demands, examine how willing he is to cooperate, and determine whether he is using the guilt you may feel about being able-bodied to manipulate you.

Timing of demands and needs. Dependency and control conflicts are evident whenever your care recipient's needs are consistently ill-timed. It's not just that his needs fail to fit into your schedule; they intensify at the worst possible times. One woman noticed after providing care for her disabled husband for a few years that his crises almost always coincided with important family functions and events: graduations, bar mitzvahs, engagements, baby showers. His message, "I need you now!"—whether spoken aloud or just implied—caused the caregiver to come running. The recipient, not she, was determining what happened and when it happened.

Unwillingness to cooperate. A care recipient can maneuver for control by refusing to cooperate. Some individuals refuse to take their medications. Others fail to perform required exercises or to help themselves in other ways. One fifty-five-year-old had suffered a mild traumatic brain injury which made him subject to seizures. Although the seizures could be controlled by medication, he steadfastly refused to take it. His refusals raised the anxiety level of his family; that was his way of maintaining control.

Manipulation through guilt. The care recipient may exert control by evoking guilty feelings in his caregiver for not being completely available. Whether or not he utters the words "Don't leave me!", the message, nevertheless, hangs in the air. So powerful may this message be that the caregiver becomes unable to take care of anything but her recipient's needs. More than one caregiver has become ill because of the resultant self-neglect.

Caregiver Dependency

Caregivers themselves may subtly surrender control to the care recipient. Do any of the following warning signs describe your attitudes or behavior?

The need to succeed. Some caregivers feel compelled to accomplish the impossible. In one case, two parents refused to accept the fact that their special needs child required medication. Determined that love and stimulation were all that he needed to succeed in school, they showered him with affection and exhausted themselves entertaining him. Instead of solving his problem, however, they created a new one: the boy learned to manipulate his parents and became a behavior problem in school. Their extraordinary efforts put him in a position of absolute control.

Excessive responsiveness. The tendency to respond too quickly to every demand, need, and crisis is closely tied to the need to succeed. Sometimes out of real concern and sometimes out of guilt, family caregivers fail to maintain perspective and distance. When this happens, they surrender control to their charge. By contrast, professional caregivers learn to pace themselves. For example, the families of hospitalized patients often expect hospital staff to respond instantly, regardless of the urgency of the need. "My son pressed the button to call the nurse," one parent complained, "and it took her two full minutes to arrive!" The nurse, knowing the patient was not in any serious danger and aware that the urgency of his needs tended to increase whenever his parents visited, did not assign the man's call a high priority. She had many patients to care for, and one of the skills she had acquired as a nurse was knowing how to gauge the urgency of the calls she received.

Take a few moments to complete the following checklist. It is designed to help you identify dependency and control conflicts in your caregiving relationship.

Caregiver Checklist: Who's in Control?

Directions: Please respond to each of the questions below by circling Y for *yes* or N for *no*.

1. Within the past week, I found myself re-arranging my schedule on short notice to meet nonessential needs of my care recipient.
   Y N

2. When I think carefully about events that have transpired over the last several months, I realize that my care recipient's crises have coincided with important events in my life or my family's.   Y N

3. Even though my care recipient is not critically ill, I sometimes put off doing things I would enjoy (going to dinner with a friend, for example) because he may need me.
   Y N

4. I feel so sorry for my care recipient that I feel guilty enjoying anything.   Y N

5. It seems the harder I work to provide loving care, the more my care recipient expects of me.   Y N

6. If I am unavailable, my care recipient creates crises to force others to take care of him.   Y N

7. No matter what the doctor says, my superior and consistent care will make my recipient better.   Y N

8. Sometimes my care recipient doesn't do what he is told, or fails to make an honest effort to help himself.   Y N

9. When my care recipient feels anxious or depressed, I find myself feeling that way, too.   Y   N

10. I sometimes refuse offers of help because I am convinced no one else can provide the same level and quality of care that I provide.   Y   N

Scoring: Give yourself one point for every Y you circled. If you scored 5 or above on the quiz, it's likely that dependency and control conflicts are adversely affecting your relationship with your care recipient.

Caregiver and Care Recipient Roles

Like lovers, business partners, or athletes in a competition, caregivers and care recipients share a reciprocal relationship, in which each person's behavior shapes the other's. Reciprocal roles can be mutually rewarding or frustrating. Hence, the relationship between caregivers and their charges is fraught with possibilities for joy and satisfaction, as well as sadness and frustration. By understanding the nature of the two roles, you will see why this potential exists.

Formally defined, a role is a collection of behaviors associated with a particular position in a group. If you have ever led a business team or taught a class, you know what the role of leader involves. Leaders motivate, plan, organize, and oversee the implementation of ideas. Those are the behaviors people expect of them. Subordinates may play a variety of roles. Some complement and reinforce the group's efforts, others provide needed information. Still others relieve tension, while a few subordinates may block or undermine the group's efforts, perhaps because they have a gripe or a hidden agenda.

We play many roles simultaneously. You may be a wife, a daughter, a mother, a sibling, a friend. You have likely become quite skilled at "wearing different hats" depending on the situation you're in. Each time you "change hats," you behave in ways called for by the role you are playing at the moment.

The behaviors expected of caregivers and care recipients are different, but the roles are always interdependent. Some of the ways that caregivers and care recipients shape each other's behavior are described in the table below. Note that for the purposes of this table, we are making two assumptions. First, we are assuming that the care recipient is capable of cooperating with the caregiver. We realize that in some cases the care recipient may be unable to perform any of the behaviors described. (This happens when care recipients are extremely young, extremely old, or completely incapacitated.) Second, we are assuming the existence of a fundamentally sound relationship between the two parties.

The Reciprocal Roles of Caregiver and Care Recipient

Representative Caregiver Behaviors	Representative Care Recipient Behaviors
Identify needs of care recipient and find ways to satisfy them	Identify own needs and make it possible for caregiver to help satisfy them; as required, let caregiver know how to satisfy those needs
Gather needed information about care recipient's condition	Provide needed information for caregiver or facilitate access to that information
Provide help willingly	Accept help graciously
Seek reassurance that the help being provided is, indeed, what is needed	Reassure caregiver that the help being provided is needed
Maintain communication about "how things are going"	Maintain communication about "how things are going"
Set boundaries so that the burdens of caregiving don't become overwhelming	Accept boundaries set by caregiver
Interact with care recipient's health-care providers to ensure cooperation	Encourage and facilitate interaction between caregiver and health-care providers
Seek outside help as needed	Accept outside help when the caregiver has reached the limit of her capabilities

As this table suggests, success in the caregiving relationship depends on both parties' willingness to cooperate. If the recipient is unable or unwilling to do his part, the burdens on the caregiver— both physical and emotional—are increased tremendously.

Troubleshooting

When your caregiving relationship is flawed, you must change the contract that exists between the two of you. Most likely, you will find that expectations, rights, and responsibilities are either unclear or skewed in favor of the care recipient. For example, the contract may give the care recipient an almost unlimited right to ask for help, even with tasks he is perfectly capable of performing himself.

If your care recipient is able to participate in revising the terms of the contract, share the responsibility. Use the worksheet on the following pages as a guide.

If your care recipient is unable to participate in this activity, at least be clear in your own mind about what you are willing to do, and what, if anything, needs to change.

If you are a member of a caregiver support group, we recommend that you use the following worksheet as a basis for a structured group activity.

Caregiving Contract Worksheet

Directions: You and your care recipient should cooperate in responding to the following items.

I. Caregiver's Rights

As the caregiver in this relationship, I now have the following rights (for example, the right to take coffee breaks):

1. _____

2. _____

3. _____

As the caregiver in this relationship, I wish to add the following rights:

1. _____

2. _____

3. _____

II. Caregiver's Responsibilities

As the caregiver in this relationship, I now have the following responsibilities (for example, administering a daily sponge bath):

1. _____

2. _____

3. _____

As the caregiver in this relationship, I wish to alter my responsibilities as follows:

1. _____

2. _____

3. _____

III. Care Recipient's Rights

The care recipient in this relationship now has the following rights (for example, the right to request help at any time).

1. _____

2. _____

3. _____

The care recipient's rights will be expanded or limited as follows:

1. _____

2. _____

3. _____

IV. Care Recipient's Responsibilities

The care recipient in this relationship now has the following responsibilities (for example, he is responsible for dressing himself in the morning).

1. _____

2. _____

3. _____

The care recipient's responsibilities will be expanded or limited as follows:

1. _____

2. _____

3. _____

Although dependency and control issues often can be resolved by revising the contract between caregiver and care recipient, diligence is required to ensure that these conflicts do not reappear. Because the care recipient is likely to be preoccupied with his own condition, we recommend that you assume responsibility for observing what is going on between the two of you. At any indication of a problem, take steps to correct the situation. Examine your motives. Look at those of your care recipient. If possible, talk about what's happening.

Principles and Paradoxes of the Caregiving Relationship

The following principles may seem paradoxical because they run counter to the usual view of things. Nevertheless, they offer a useful way of thinking about the relationship.

To Accept Help Is an Act of Generosity

Have you ever tried to help someone who was in need, only to have your offer rejected? If so, you know how upsetting the experience can be. When someone refuses your offer in a misguided effort to remain independent, you feel hurt and rejected. On the other hand, when a care recipient accepts your offer, you feel appreciated.

Consider Marjorie's case. She was the only child of an elderly widow who lived two hours away from her. For many years, occasional visits were sufficient for Marjorie to provide the care that was needed. She would arrive, see to her mother's physical, social, and emotional needs, and help out with a few tasks around the house. During those years, each visit was highlighted by a pleasant outing. Over time, however, the visits took on a different tone; they became less social and more like social work. As Marjorie's mother began failing and her ability to walk diminished, she was reluctant to venture out of the house. The pleasant outings came to an end. Marjorie also noted that her mother had begun withdrawing from friends and neighbors, refusing to answer the phone, and being curt and short-tempered if she did. Her mother also suffered from occasional incontinence, for which she refused to seek help. Marjorie noted that this reinforced her mother's tendency to isolate herself.

Eventually it became clear that the elderly woman's deteriorating physical and emotional condition was making it impossible for her to continue to live on her own. She rarely cooked, because she could no longer remember how, and she was subsisting on crackers, yogurt, ice cream, and milk. Had it not been for the pre-cooked meals Marjorie brought to her, the elderly woman would have had no hot meals at all. Her home was no longer clean—she had been a meticulous homemaker—and reeked of urine. Furthermore, in an attempt to manage the unpleasant consequences of her incontinence, Marjorie's mother had taken actions that resulted in sewage blockages, which cost many hundreds of dollars to fix. The house was deteriorating along with the older woman's physical and emotional health. In addition to feeding her mother and cleaning for her, Marjorie arranged for home repairs. Marjorie said sadly, "I feel like I keep putting my fingers in a dike. But I'm running out of fingers."

Marjorie had only a few alternative solutions. One was to hire people who would come into the home and tend to her mother's needs and the tasks of day-to-day living. When she raised that possibility, her mother flatly refused to consider it. Another option was to have her mother live with Marjorie and her family. The third was to have her mother enter a nursing home. To each of these suggestions, her mother reacted with screams of protest. "I'm in charge of my life!" she raged. "Just leave me alone!"

Marjorie reported that such responses made her feel inconsequential and worthless, like a little girl who wanted to help but whose efforts and good will were rather cruelly rejected. "My mother may not know it," she said at the time, "but her refusals to accept help are devastating." Marjorie found that her mother's refusal to acknowledge her need for greater help complicated Marjorie's own life tremendously, burdening her in ways that she did not feel were fair or necessary. Whatever the reasons for the elderly woman's behavior, it was injurious not only to herself, but to her daughter, too. It took Marjorie many months to come to terms with her sadness and anger.

To Give Help Can Be a Selfish Act

An overly solicitous caregiver may actually retard her care recipient's progress by fostering dependency while serving her own need to be needed. Any parent who has had a child in nursery school is familiar with this dynamic. "Drop-off time" in many nursery schools is often very distressing, as some mothers have more difficulty separating from their children than their youngsters do in separating from them. Feeling empty and unneeded without a dependent child in tow, some mothers react to their children's movement toward autonomy with sadness and anxiety. Sensing their mothers' discomfort and distress, these children become anxious themselves, and lose confidence in their ability to function on their own.

Caregivers may foster dependency in similar ways and for much the same reason. Needing to be needed, they undermine the care recipient's efforts to regain lost capabilities.

Sometimes the caregiver's motives are sinister. In one instance, an errant husband actually encouraged his wife's fear of leaving her home. (She suffered from a psychological condition called agoraphobia.) His reason, however, had more to do with his love affairs than with his spouse's well-being. By the time she arrived at our office, this woman had seen scores of physicians. She literally brought a small satchel of medications with her to the first meeting, declaring that she had become so tired of being sick and taking medication that she would rather die. As her solicitous husband patiently described her emotional problems, he seemed the very picture of concern. But as our work soon revealed, his motivations were almost entirely selfish.

The goal of the caregiver ought to be the same as that of any other nurturing authority: to promote independence and maximize the care recipient's ability to function independently.

Providing Help Can Be Gratifying Even If It Means a Lot of Work

Giving help carries its own rewards. When a person in your life needs care, you have the choice of providing help yourself, or allowing others to assume the burden of caregiving. By opting out, you preserve the pace and rhythm of your life as you have structured it. Your work, home life, and social life remain unchanged. By contrast, providing care requires that your life be disrupted to some degree, sometimes to a very large degree. Comfortable routines must be abandoned. The unspoken rules governing family life must be revised. Although this does involve personal sacrifice, the choice to provide care may enhance a sense of usefulness and add a special dimension to an already caring relationship. As one young woman said, "I went into this dreading every minute of it, but I soon learned that few things I do are more rewarding".

It Takes a Strong Person to Relinquish Control

Most people believe that if you play according to the rules, take care of yourself, and do the right thing, nothing bad will befall you. When an accident occurs, illness strikes, or a longed-for child is born severely damaged, our sense of rightness and order is seriously challenged. "Why me?" asked one woman whose husband was injured in a freak auto accident. "Why couldn't he have left five minutes later?" (However, the very term "accident" implies a loss of control or the effects of a random event, and asking that question in such a context never helps.) Both caregiver and care recipient are contending with forces over which they may have little or no control, and they both may feel weak, helpless, and angry at the unfairness of it all. Giving and receiving care under these circumstances is fraught with sorrow and frustration, which must be acknowledged and resolved.

Setting Boundaries Gives Greater Freedom

Out of love and compassion, most caregivers feel an initial reluctance to set limits. They want to be so completely available to their care recipient that they put aside all other priorities, believing they are doing the right thing. Eventually, most come to realize that every relationship needs limits. Caregivers who make themselves too available eventually wind up filled with resentment. Since care recipients are more likely to feel respected when treated as able-bodied, if they can to do things for themselves, they should be expected to do so.

Because being a caregiver is just one of the many roles you play, it should not become all-consuming. By setting limits and boundaries, you protect your own interests while meeting the needs of the person for whom you provide care.

CHAPTER THREE

UNTHINKABLE THOUGHTS AND UNACCEPTABLE FEELINGS: COMING TO TERMS WITH GIVING AND RECEIVING CARE

You cannot avoid having strong reactions to becoming a caregiver or a care recipient. This chapter is about the importance of recognizing and accepting these reactions and their associated feelings, especially negative ones, such as anger and resentment. Failure to do so can greatly interfere with your ability to give or accept help.

"I've got to see you this morning!" Sylvia cried into the telephone when her therapist returned her five A.M. call. "Something terrible's happened!" An eight o'clock appointment was arranged. Sylvia arrived at the office promptly. By the time she got there, she was a little calmer. "Last night after dinner, when my mother refused to eat again, I got so angry, I slapped her—in the face!" she blurted out, embarrassed. "And then I cursed her! She looked so shocked! Then she cried and cried. I felt awful! But it's even worse. After a while she calmed down. I thought I'd calmed down, too." She paused. "But when I finally went to sleep, I had awful nightmares. I don't remember them all, but in one I was scratching at her face with my fingernails! She was screaming in pain! And I was crying and laughing! Then I woke up. I'm afraid I'm going to hurt her more! That's when I called you."

Sylvia's behavior and her dream indicated something needed to be done right away. Her therapist persuaded her to make arrangements for a relative to take over her mother's care for a few days; then Sylvia made longer-term plans to share the burden of her mother's care and to put her own life back in balance.

Caregivers' Feelings

Becoming a caregiver requires many adjustments from the outset. Some caregivers may need to leave a job. Others must rearrange their homes and turn their familiar world topsy-turvy. Often, their social life disappears, as friends withdraw because of their own discomfort, thereby depriving the caregiver of much-needed support. "Sometimes, the silence is deafening," one woman observed.

Caregivers cannot help having emotional reactions. During the initial period of fear and uncertainty they may feel overwhelmed by all they must learn to do. As their confidence grows, other feelings, such as anger and resentment, may begin to emerge. For Sylvia, as with many caregivers, acknowledging these negative feelings is very uncomfortable. Nevertheless it is necessary to do so.

The Importance of Knowing How You Feel

Being in touch with your feelings is essential for three crucial reasons.

1. *Unacknowledged feelings can lead to bad decisions.* Sometimes it is necessary to make difficult and painful decisions, such as institutionalizing a special needs child, putting an elderly parent in a nursing home, or authorizing a "do-not-resuscitate" order for a terminally ill spouse. In such cases, if you are not absolutely clear about your own feelings, you may make inappropriate decisions.

Many years ago, one of the authors took a group of college students on a field trip to a state school for the retarded. The social worker conducting the tour spoke with pride of a devoted parent who made the long trip to the school each week to visit her profoundly retarded son, despite the fact that he was incapable of recognizing her. One astute student commented that the mother sounded motivated more by guilt than by love. Although the social worker bristled, the student was correct. While the parent had recognized the need to institutionalize her son, she had been unable to come to terms with her guilt at doing so.

2. *Clear-headedness is required to trust your own judgment.* One mother of a cerebral-palsied child resisted the advice of well-meaning professionals to institutionalize her daughter as an infant and go on with her own life. The mother correctly determined that home care was both appropriate and manageable. Unburdened by guilt or anger, she was able to raise her child to be a successful and independent adult.

The same principle applies when you are providing care for an elderly person. Decisions about surgery, placement in a nursing home, and similar matters demand a clear head. Care alternatives can be explored freely only in the absence of guilt and rage. Although professionals can be consulted to obtain an objective perspective, they may have their own agendas and biases, and their opinions should not be regarded as final. This is especially true when their opinions go against your own inclinations. Furthermore, professional advisors do not have to live with the consequences of the decisions they recommend. When one eighty-five-year-old woman with mid-stage Alzheimer's was diagnosed with ovarian cancer, her oncologist recommended surgery. The family considered his recommendation and flatly rejected it. They knew her wishes, and found unconscionable the prospect of painful and intrusive treatment for a woman too impaired to understand what was happening. She died peacefully one week later, still intact enough to recognize the people who visited her in her final days.

3. *Knowing your feelings can help you cope.* Rather than viewing them as something to fear and conceal, you can use your feelings like gauges on your car's instrument panel—as indicators of what's going on "beneath the hood." Your feelings can help you determine where "maintenance work" needs to be done. Sam's story is a case in point. For most of his life Sam had been regarded as a chronic complainer. Always clear about how he felt, if something bothered him, he made no secret of it. When Sarah, his wife of many years, began showing signs of memory loss, he was distressed. However, he promptly had her evaluated by a neurologist. Although shaken and depressed by Sarah's diagnosis of dementia, he

arranged for a home-health aide to lighten his load, and devoted himself to her care. He was not receptive to support groups, but the loving woman who came to clean and prepare meals also served as a source of emotional support. Sam remained caring and attentive until Sarah's death several years later. After a period of mourning, he worked through his feelings of loss. Today, at eighty-nine, he plays bridge, has a woman companion, and retains his sense of humor. Because Sam had been able to acknowledge his sadness and frustration, he was able to ask for the help he needed.

How We Learn to Discount Unwanted Feelings

Although being in touch with your feelings sounds as if it should be as natural as breathing, many people, caregivers included, are often quite unable to access their "inner life," especially when the feelings involved are viewed as unacceptable. The tendency to discount feelings originates in childhood. Consider the following conversation between a grandmother and her granddaughter, who had just become a big sister. The grandmother asked the child how she liked her new brother. "I hate him!" her granddaughter replied. "No you don't," said Grandma. "You love him. You don't know how lucky you are to have a little brother!" But the child knows she doesn't love her brother and that she is feeling hurt and angry at all the attention he gets. Nevertheless, she wants her grandma to love her, so she says nothing in response to grandma's admonition. Instead, she vents her anger on her baby brother in hugs that hurt and in outbursts of temper that seem to come from nowhere. If this child is typical, she will feel confused and guilty about feeling so angry, and is also likely to be branded a "jealous sibling" by unthinking adults.

Adults cope similarly. When "unacceptable" feelings can't be expressed directly, they show up indirectly as angry words that slip out, as impatience that confuses and hurts, as headaches that seem to have no clear source, and as murderous or vengeful thoughts.

Why Caregiving Evokes Strong Negative Feelings

Caregivers are often powerless to alter the realities of their care recipient's condition and its impact on their lives. Here are several unavoidable "facts of life" that family caregivers invariably must face:

1. *Daily frustrations.* Almost any caregiving task, however unpleasant, can be tolerated for a short time. However, when repeated day in and day out, it can quickly become intolerable. Each new day, instead of being filled with promise in the usual hopeful sense, is filled with the promise of a known unpleasantness. Over time, the resultant tension, if ignored, can reach devastating and destructive levels. One mother, the sole caregiver of a profoundly retarded child, described every day as a living hell, and felt that the death of her child would be far less painful for her to bear than the interminable torture of her daily caregiving.

2. *Limitations on personal activities and family life.* Sheryl has two children. One of them was born with a disorder that makes it impossible for him to relate to others in a normal way. Asked about her experience, this is what she said:

   "Jeremy is almost four now, and we still don't have a definitive diagnosis! He is definitely not autistic, but he is a terror at home! For some reason, at times he just explodes," she fumed. "We've taken Jeremy to the best children's hospitals in the country. We've seen doctor after doctor! Attention deficit disorder, autism, pervasive developmental disorder—everybody has an opinion, but nobody knows what to do for him! Sometimes, he's such a sweetheart! He's such a good-hearted kid. But he can be the world's greatest pain in the butt! I've learned, though," Sheryl continued. "Now I'm grateful for little things. When I can go to the supermarket and spend twenty minutes shopping without a scene I'm very grateful for that."

Sheryl's comments speak not only to limitations on caregivers' personal and family life, but to other adaptations as well. They must learn to lower their expectations, to be grateful for what they once thought they could take for granted.

The family of a severely autistic child may be unable to enjoy dinner at a restaurant, let alone go on a vacation. Siblings may be unable to invite friends to the house. Adult children of a parent suffering from dementia may be so preoccupied that even if they do find time to socialize, they may be unable to relax and enjoy themselves. When limitations are expected, and when there are joys to balance the sacrifice (for example, when a normal child is born), the impact of these restrictions is generally tolerable. But when limitations aren't accompanied by any pleasure, they can quickly become suffocating. Feelings are heightened when family members other than the caregiver are affected. A disturbed child's siblings, for example, may themselves then burden the already-stressed care provider with their own frustration and unhappiness.

3. *Neglect of physical needs.* Because of the time and energy demanded by the care recipient, caregivers may neglect their own needs. The effects of fatigue and poor eating habits tend to be cumulative. Over time, the caregiver's own coping resources may become severely compromised, resulting in depression and erratic behavior.

4. *Neglect of social needs.* As mentioned earlier, caregivers may be unable to fulfill their own social needs because of the discomfort of friends who don't know what to say or do. When someone dies, there are clear rituals that guide friends and family in providing comfort to the bereaved. We sit shiva, attend a wake, or go to the funeral. No such rituals exist to provide comfort to individuals whose loved one has become disabled, or to console a woman who has given birth to a retarded child.

5. *Long-term caregiving.* Sometimes caregiving continues over many years, as with a chronic illness, or the birth of a disabled child who will need lifetime care. The potential for personal distress and disrupted family relationships in situations like these is far greater than when there is an end in sight.

Mike and Terry's case illustrate this fact. Their first child, Celeste, was born brain damaged, and would never be capable of living on her own. As the years passed and Celeste approached adulthood, provision for her long-term care became increasingly problematic. Mike and Terry's marriage, stressed for many years, began to falter, and they eventually divorced.

6. *Lack of choice.* As we explained in chapter 1, there are many reasons why individuals become caregivers, some healthier than others. However, when the primary reason is that there is no other logical choice, the potential for resentment is far greater than when the caregiving has been chosen, regardless of the underlying motivation.

7. *Death of a fantasy.* When a special needs child is born, the parents must cope not only with the prospect of lifelong caregiving, but with grief and the guilt over the loss of the

expected normal child. Similar reactions occur when a spouse or partner becomes permanently disabled. Although the marriage vows include the phrase "in sickness and in health," the assumption is almost always that the couple will enjoy many years of mutual good health. In coping with this abrupt and unexpected transition, the caregiver must mourn and come to terms with the "death" of an anticipated future.

In the late 1990s, Sally was living well. Her husband was a highly successful physician looking forward to earnings approaching $200,000 per year at a prestigious teaching hospital. Then, one Sunday afternoon, everything changed. As Sally, her husband, and their young child were driving to a relative's home, a teenage girl, newly licensed, made a serious error of judgment on a crowded expressway. The awful accident that followed caused injuries to everyone in the family, and left Sally's husband permanently impaired. He suffered not only physical injuries resulting in chronic back pain, but a traumatic brain injury that left him unable to continue working as a physician. Sally was grieved by her loss, and saddened by her own injuries and those of her husband and child. She uttered the same question over and over again in different forms: "Why me? Why did this have to happen to me? We worked hard to get where we were! My husband had just begun coming into his own. He was well respected. Our future held the rewards that had been so long in coming. And now this! It's just so damned unfair!"

8. *Lack of gratitude.* Care recipients are often ungrateful. One elderly care recipient complained endlessly about the lack of variety of the food in his nursing home. His negative attitude alienated many people and was especially painful to his daughter, who had been so pleased when she finally found an attractive facility that was well suited to his needs and interests.

9. *Facing the realities of a care recipient's condition.* The shock of facing unwanted realities may also evoke strong feelings. When Barbara, the adult child of an Alzheimer's patient, discovered that her mother no longer recognized her, she became depressed. In discussing her reaction, she observed, "Mom has no idea who I am. I've truly lost my mother and am now paying visits to a total stranger. I still visit weekly to be sure she is being cared for properly, but in many ways it's harder to take than if she had actually died."

Burying Negative Feelings

There are four reasons why accepting negative feelings is so difficult. They are as follows:

1. *Need for approval.* We sometimes don't say what we feel because of the fear of disapproval. However, when we "hide out" from others often enough and with enough skill, we end up "hiding out" from ourselves. As a result, we lose touch with our feelings.

2. *Violation of family rules.* Some families have unspoken rules against acknowledging and sharing feelings. Consider the following story. Alberto, married for fifty-two years to Juanita, was a devoted husband. His own history included periodic episodes of depression, which had been carefully hidden from his three daughters. When Juanita began showing signs of memory loss, Alberto kept the problem to himself and pretended that nothing was wrong. He gradually assumed all the household responsibilities, saying nothing until the day Juanita tried to put a roll of toilet paper into the kitchen paper towel holder. At that point, he fell apart, and told his oldest daughter that he could not go on. Within days, he became so depressed that he required hospitalization.

3. *Gratitude.* When a patient is difficult, the caregiver feels fully justified in being angry and frustrated. However, pleasant and grateful patients can pose just as serious a problem. Suppose you were to spend every Saturday visiting your ailing mother and that she was extremely grateful. Although you might resent giving up your Saturdays, her appreciation would undermine your comfort with your reaction. Any resentment you might feel would seem wrong.

Care recipients may use gratitude to manipulate their caregivers by inducing guilt. The needy spouse who declares you the most important person in her world, or the only stable person she can count on, places you in an impossible position. Attending to your own needs, should they conflict with her demands, seems heartless and cruel. This manipulation can go on for years, and can involve not only the primary caregiver but other family members as well.

4. *Belief in the power of thoughts.* Some caregivers believe that just having strong negative feelings, even if they never act on them, is bad. For them, the primitive belief that wishes have power, that just thinking something can make it come true, never fully disappears. This fear, irrational though it is,

inhibits their ability to acknowledge their negative feelings and fantasies.

Tuning In to Your Feelings

People differ in how easily they can acknowledge their feelings. As a rule, because of their social conditioning, women are more comfortable discussing their feelings than men are, and they have more emotional outlets available to them. If you are having difficulty accessing your feelings about caregiving, you will find the following suggestions helpful.

Tune in to your body. When people say that they don't "feel well," they may be translating an emotional state into a physical one. Children generally have difficulty expressing feelings in words, and so tend to experience physical symptoms. David, the twelve-year-old "hidden caregiver" of a depressed parent, was overwhelmed by his self-imposed responsibility to "make Daddy happy." He developed recurrent headaches and complained often about not feeling well, even though he was obviously not physically ill. Unable to articulate distress at his inappropriate role, he let his body speak for him. His symptoms also provided temporary relief from his caregiving activities, forcing him to lie down and have his mother take care of him.

Take note of any inclination on your part to convert emotional distress into physical symptoms. If you develop symptoms such as headaches or exhaustion in the absence of a physical cause, look closely at what was going on when the symptoms appeared. You may be able to identify the trigger.

Respect your fantasies. Whenever you find your mind drifting off in unexpected or troubling directions, take a hard look at what is going on. One client reported that while pushing her elderly mother in her wheelchair, she imagined thrusting the chair into the path of an oncoming truck. Another caregiver fantasized about having a room all to herself, with no one to take care of, nothing to clean or organize, just the total freedom to sit in a comfortable chair, eat, and read. Yet another said, with some embarrassment, "I found myself wishing that I could get sick. Not uncomfortably sick, but sick enough for someone to have to take care of me for a change!"

Attend to unexpected behaviors. After having an argument with her mother, Janet was puzzled over the failure of her attempt to apologize. "I tried to say I was sorry, but the harder I tried, the angrier I got. I wonder now if I really felt sorry in the first place!" When things don't work out as expected, there is a good chance that you were not accurately reading your own feelings; what may have come out, instead, was what you were truly feeling. Unexpected outbursts of tears or anger send the same message. "I couldn't believe I actually threw pizza at my husband," Caryn said, with amazement. "But all of a sudden my arm seemed to have a life of its own. Actually, even though I was embarrassed, it felt good."

Although often uncomfortable, these unexpected events provide a clear message. Failure to heed them puts you at risk for loss of control.

What to Do with Feelings You've "Just Discovered"

Once you've accessed your true feelings, what should you do with them? Here are some effective ways to follow through.

1. *Writing.* You can hand-write your thoughts in a diary or type them into a computer. You can save what you've written or toss it. You can write poetry, or letters, or just use your writing to clarify your thoughts. The form is irrelevant. What matters is getting your feelings out.

2. *Grievance list.* Because it often helps to see things in writing, jot down those things about caregiving that are most distressing to you. Look carefully at each item with a focus on resolving the feelings and conflicts it reveals. For example, if one of your items suggests you need more free time for yourself, think about people you might contact for relief. If many problems seem unsolvable, consider joining a support group or organization so you can benefit from the experiences of others.

3. *Support groups.* Many hospitals and social service organizations sponsor support groups. In such a group you can talk about feelings, acquire skills, and learn about resources. You can meet other people who have themselves "been there," and who can be truly empathic. You can also learn to deal with doctors and other professionals more effectively. Depending on the particular mix of personalities and the care with which meetings are planned, some groups are more helpful than others. If you find that the first group you join isn't useful, try at least one more before giving up. The Resources section at the back of the book contains a list of organizations that sponsor groups that may meet your needs. Other sources are your care recipient's physician, friends, relatives, and even people in doctors' waiting rooms.

4. *The empty chair.* If there are things you would like to say to your care recipient but are unable to do so, try this exercise. Find a time when you can be assured of privacy. Set up two chairs, as though you were going to have a conversation. Seat yourself on one, and imagine your care recipient on the other. Talk to him as if he were actually there, using "I" statements. ("I" statements are sentences that begin with "I," such as, "I feel angry when you criticize everything that I do." They help you focus on what you are feeling. Sentences that start with "you," such as, "You make me angry when you criticize me," shift the responsibility to the other person, and are much less helpful, since you can't control someone else's behavior.) Keep talking until you've had your say. This is not a dialogue; it is your opportunity to say exactly what you want. You might feel uncomfortable initially—people don't ordinarily talk to empty chairs—but the potential for a meaningful venting of your feelings makes it worthwhile to see this through.

5. *The Internet.* The Internet can be a valuable source of support, especially if you cannot easily leave your home. There are numerous websites that focus on caregiver feelings and experiences and provide on-line support. Two of these are:

   http://www.caregiving.com/

   http://www.caregiver.org/

6. *Mental health professionals.* If you are still unable to find relief, seek out a properly licensed mental health professional for support, preferably one with caregiving experience. Seeing a therapist does not mean that you are weak or crazy, but that you are strong enough to seek help when you can't go it alone. It also means that you are unwilling to settle for less than the best you can be and feel—both for your own sake and for that of your care recipient.

The Care Recipient's Feelings

Like caregivers, care recipients often struggle with strong feelings that are difficult to acknowledge. These feelings originate in the transition from self-sufficiency to dependency. According to medical social worker Wendy Lustbader (1991), the care recipient must make many difficult adjustments. Here are the ones she identifies as critical:

1. **Accepting dependency.**

Whether the process is abrupt or gradual, the care recipient must come to terms with the fact that he is dependent on someone else for things he used to do for himself.

2. **Accepting the loss of an active life.**

The care recipient may also have to make the transition from an active life to one of little or no activity, perhaps even a life of confinement. In a society like ours that places so much emphasis on freedom and independence, being unable to come and go at will reflects a real loss.

3. **Accepting unwanted changes in relationships.**

The care recipient must redefine his relationships with others. He may also lose some relationships altogether. One man, for example, complained that his golfing partners lost interest in him as soon as he could no longer join them on the links. "They just stopped calling! It was as if I'd fallen off the face of the earth!" Another noted that some of his workmates visited him at home once or twice after he became ill, but that most of them dropped out of touch after their awkward and obviously unsatisfying visits. They actually had created problems, he observed, that were disproportionate to the comfort their visits had provided. Insensitive to the patient's needs, they had interfered with necessary activities such as resting, feeding, and bathing, and had burdened the patient with their needs to be reassured and entertained.

4. **Accepting limitations and moving on.**

Perhaps most demanding of all, care recipients must find new ways to take satisfaction in life, new ways of using remaining capabilities. For example, a talented trumpeter, whose career ended abruptly when a heart disorder was diagnosed, channeled his ability into teaching. A young woman whose hand was severed when she was pushed in front of an oncoming train became a rehabilitation counselor.

How Care Recipients Feel

Given the nature and extent of these necessary adjustments, it is not surprising that care recipients often struggle with feelings of anger, fear, depression, and frustration.

Sandy was a successful, personable, and well-liked high school teacher when she was diagnosed with multiple sclerosis (MS). "When I was diagnosed, my first reaction was denial. 'This can't be happening to me,' I said. 'This kind of thing happens to other people.' My husband and I went to four neurologists before I was convinced. Up until then, I was certain Dr. Cooper had made a terrible mistake. I remember when the diagnosis was confirmed, I felt furious and very sorry for myself. For a long time, I would not talk with anyone about it. I didn't want my family told. My mother was in her seventies. She didn't need to hear this. I wanted no one to know, not even my sister. I thought I could beat the disease. 'I won't be like all the others,' I told myself. 'I'm an educated woman. I can help myself. I can read and try alternative therapies.' It was months before I came to terms with the diagnosis. Herb [her husband] was a saint! I was really pretty unreasonable!"

Sandy, for all her struggle, is at least able to articulate her feelings clearly. It is far worse when someone can't do it directly.

How Care Recipients Express Feelings Indirectly

1. **The care recipient may reject the caregiver's offers of help.**

Juan, a man in his fifties, sustained a back injury and was left with serious and chronic pain. At times he could not even walk and was reduced to crawling around on all fours. Yet he adamantly refused his wife's offers of help, preferring to maintain the illusion that he did not need her.

2. **Some care recipients are ungrateful.**

Care recipients are often ungrateful for the help they receive. "My father rarely thanks me for anything I do for him," said one young woman. "I get so mad sometimes! The more I do, the more he expects." Her reactions are understandable, but so are her father's, who feels humiliated by having to accept help from the daughter he raised.

3. **The care recipient may become self-centered and noncommunicative.**

"She's quick to ask for what she needs," Greg said of his thirty-three-year-old wife. "But when I try to engage her in conversation about anything else, she just clams up. She's not interested in anyone but herself!" Following a botched surgery on her knee, Brenda had developed a series of physical problems and became depressed. Uncomfortable about having to depend on her husband for help, she reacted by becoming self-absorbed and withdrawn.

4. **The care recipient may become obnoxious and controlling.**

A family complained that an elderly member had become downright obnoxious. Grandma Sara, as she was called, refused to let her grandchildren sit on her bed. "I paid for this bed!" she scolded when they came to her room to visit. "Stay off it!" She pushed her family away constantly with an endless array of abusive comments. Grandma Sara's disagreeableness was her way of coping with the humiliation and anger she felt at having to depend on them for her care.

5. **The care recipient may withhold important information in order to "protect" her caregiver.**

One woman, whose elderly father had moved in with her and her family, reported that he had been admitted to the hospital with severe chest pain. She was distressed when she learned that he had been experiencing chest pain for several days. "My father never told me!" she exclaimed. "Why would he do that?" The reason, as it turned out, was that he had not wanted to burden her with still more worries about him.

This kind of behavior on the part of care recipients is not at all unusual. One man's ninety-year-old mother, who lived alone, had had an electrical power loss at her home for several hours, but had kept it a secret. Asked why she had not called, she said simply, "I didn't want to worry you. You have enough on your mind."

If your care recipient is unable to express feelings directly, you need to recognize the meaning of the person's behavior and respond to what is meant, not to what is said or done. By being diligent about respecting your own feelings and those of your recipient, your ability to provide appropriate and sensitive care will be enhanced immeasurably.

PART TWO

COPING AS A CAREGIVER

Family caregivers typically contend with stress and frustration as they struggle to meet the needs of their care recipients while taking care of their own lives. They must juggle homemaking, work, and child-care responsibilities, while also meeting personal and social needs and obligations.

This part of the book focuses on the challenges faced by caregivers. We show you how to manage the feelings evoked by caregiving and suggest ways of working cooperatively with family members, health-care professionals, and others. We also offer ways of proceeding when difficulties arise.

The problems posed by special caregiving situations are addressed in this part of the book, too. What is the best way of managing the situation when a care recipient isn't identified as such? Or is mentally ill? Or is a special needs child? Or lives far away from the caregiver? For those who provide care for a person who is elderly or terminally ill, chapter 11 discusses coping with death. Chapter 12 on how to find and select a caregiver support group explains how to make the most of this valuable resource.

CHAPTER FOUR

CAREGIVER BURNOUT

In this chapter we discuss the prevention and treatment of caregiver burnout. You will learn why it occurs, how to recognize its warning signs, and how to prevent it.

When caregivers fail to acknowledge and reduce the chronic stresses they are under, the quality of caregiving drops. As they struggle to cope, their physical and mental health may deteriorate, and their careers and relationships may suffer. Under extreme stress, they may even abuse their care recipients. In fact, abuse of one group of care recipients, the elderly, is so widespread that it is considered a national major health issue. The National Center for Elder Abuse reported, in a recent survey, that there are between 820,000 and 1,800,000 abused elders in the United States. However, this problem is not limited to the elderly: all care recipients can become targets. Even if the situation does not deteriorate to this level, the stressed-out caregiver cannot provide quality care.

Recognizing Caregiver Burnout

Burnout is most likely to occur when caregivers fail to recognize the toll their hard work is taking on them. Overburdened, frustrated, and isolated, they allow feelings to simmer inside, unaware of their urgent need for relief.

Care recipients may inadvertently contribute to this problem, since it's not unusual for pain, depression, and deteriorating physical health to result in negative personality changes. When formerly cooperative and pleasant people become insensitive, demanding, and unpleasant, additional stresses are created for the already overburdened caregiver.

The Nature of Burnout

The word "burnout" is a wonderful metaphor, suggesting a candle that, for a time, provides both light and warmth. When a candle burns too brightly or too rapidly—when the caregiver, in other words, cares too much, tries too hard, and neglects herself—the candle eventually burns itself out.

This word is often applied to professionals such as teachers, social workers, and nurses, who grow tired of facing the same problems and confronting the same anguish. They exhaust themselves contending with inadequate resources, faceless bureaucracies, and appalling rudeness. If they don't take breaks from their duties or find other ways to relieve their constant stress, they run the risk of becoming cynical, cold, angry, or worse. Many human service workers leave their jobs after several years to avoid inflicting damage on the very people they originally set out to help.

Although family caregivers run the same risks, they cannot simply quit. Many carry on long after caregiving has ceased to be even tolerable. Said one woman while trying to express what she felt after many years of caring for her disabled spouse, "I remember being enthusiastic. I used to think about Knute Rockne's remark, 'When the going gets tough, the tough get going.' Now, I guess I'm not so tough anymore. I'm just out of steam."

Here is an exercise that will familiarize you with the warning signs of burnout, and help you determine whether you are at risk:

Warning Signs of Caregiver Burnout

Directions: Please respond to each item by circling Y for yes or N for no.

1. I feel sad and "down" more often than is usual for me.
   Y N

2. Lately, I am doing fewer and fewer of the things I enjoy.
   Y N

3. I often feel overwhelmed and pressured. Y N

4. I feel very alone much of the time. Y N

5. I often cry. Y N

6. I prefer not to talk about my stresses or problems with others. Y N

7. I sometimes fear my anger will get out of control.
Y N

8. I react strongly to little annoyances. Y N

9. I'm afraid I'll do something to injure my care recipient.
Y N

10. I resent it when other people have a good time.
Y N

11. I feel "edgy" much of the time. Y N

12. I often feel something terrible is about to happen.
Y N

We have grouped the warning signs of impending burnout into five main categories. Your "yes" responses indicate your most vulnerable areas. Although often frightening, symptoms of impending burnout are not enemies to be medicated away or fought. They are your allies, clear signals to yourself that you need a break, and that changes in caregiving arrangements must be made. After a review of these warning signs, we will discuss why burnout occurs, how to cope with it, and ways to prevent it from happening.

1. **Warning Sign One: Depression (Items 1, 2, 5)**
One sure sign that you are struggling as a caregiver is that you are not feeling happy. "How can I feel happy when I have all this responsibility?" you might very well ask. True, but there is a difference between sadness and depression. No one can expect to feel happy all the time. And certainly your circumstances can account for your feeling sad, at least sometimes. However, something is very wrong if you find yourself crying and feeling "down" often, if you are unable to find time for any of the activities you enjoy doing, or if you are unable to muster the energy to get out of bed in the morning. Any of these is a warning sign of depression.

2. **Warning Sign Two: Isolation (Items 4, 6)**
Friends and family can offer the support that balances the responsibilities of caregiving. Without emotional refueling, your own resources will rapidly become depleted. Dropping out of touch, failing to return calls, and declining invitations are sure signs that you are in trouble.

3. Warning Sign Three: Anxiety (Items 3, 11, 12)

Anxiety is often expressed in physical symptoms such as muscle tension and shortness of breath, emotional symptoms (e.g., feeling that something awful is going to happen), or cognitive symptoms (e.g., feeling disorganized and distracted). Anxious caregivers are likely to be inattentive and to make mistakes. If your anxiety level is interfering with your caregiving, you must take steps to calm yourself down.

4. Warning Sign Four: Irritability (Items 8, 10)

Caregivers who are approaching burnout are impatient with everyone. The normal behaviors of children, for example, may be enough to set them off. When shopping, they may become irritated with clerks and checkout people. Stressed out and pressured, such caregivers have no tolerance for unavoidable frustrations.

5. Warning Sign Five: Anger (Items 7, 9)

All caregivers feel angry at times. However, when even mild forms of anger, such as annoyance, become chronic, it is time to take stock of what's going on. If unchecked, annoyance can escalate to rage, and caregiving will certainly be jeopardized.

Understanding Burnout

Why does burnout occur? There are two sets of reasons. Some of them have to do with the caregiver, others with the recipient.

Problems Originating with the Caregiver

1. Failure to Respect Needs

Why don't family caregivers seek relief before burning out? There are several reasons. In chapter 2, we discussed the relationship between caregivers and care recipients. We stressed the crucial importance of a clear contract, with well-defined rights and responsibilities. The purpose of this contract is to ensure that the needs of both caregiver and care recipient are respected. However, even having a good contract is not sufficient if either party ignores its terms. Many caregivers do not respect their needs, set limits, or take needed breaks. To save money, or out of a misguided sense that they alone can provide adequate care, they may:

- Decline to accept help from family members
- Resist the idea of adult day care or other forms of relief

- Fail to use respite care services such as home companions or visiting nurses

Caregivers who make these errors essentially give up their lives. Sometimes they do not even take the time to read the newspaper. They stop doing what they enjoy and spend virtually all their time on caregiving. If this description fits you, please read and think about the following Caregiver's Bill of Rights:

Caregiver's Bill of Rights

As a caregiver, I have the right . . .

- To take care of myself—to rest when I'm tired, to eat well, to take breaks from caregiving when I need them
- To recognize the limits of my own endurance and strength
- To seek help from family, involved parties, and the community at large
- To socialize, to maintain my interests, and to do the things I enjoy
- To acknowledge my feelings, whether positive or negative, including frustration, anger, and depression, and to express them constructively
- To take pride in the valuable work I do, and to applaud the courage and inventiveness it takes to meet the needs of my care recipient

2. Failure to Express Negative Feelings

Family caregivers often fail to acknowledge and talk about negative feelings when "little things" go wrong. As we observed in chapter 3, often they do not even acknowledge such feelings to themselves. For example, one young woman reported that her son, who suffered from attention deficit disorder (ADD), had been rejected by most of his peers. Nevertheless, the boy insisted on begging them to come to his home to play. He bribed them with gifts and outlandish promises about what they would do and where they would go. When he became sullen in response to the many rejections he received, his mother was more angry than sympathetic. Because she felt guilty about her anger, she couldn't imagine sharing it with her son. "How could I?" she asked. "He was already devastated." Nevertheless, had she spoken with her son, she would have not only discharged her negative feelings but could have helped him to cope more effectively.

67

3. **Failure to Confront Others**

Even when family caregivers feel unfairly burdened, most do not insist on help from others. Many, wanting to maintain peaceful and harmonious relationships, are hesitant to assert themselves and confront uncooperative family members. "If I get angry with my brother, I'll hurt his feelings," said one woman who provided round-the-clock care for their ailing father. "He'll be upset, and that won't make anything better!" People who are afraid to ask for reasonable cooperation from others may not even be aware of their anger and resentment. However, these feelings do not disappear. Instead, as we said in chapter 3, such feelings almost always find destructive ways of making themselves felt. Although confrontation is seldom pleasant, in the long run its benefits outweigh its risks.

Problems Originating with the Care Recipient

So far, we've spoken about how the caregiver's behavior contributes to burnout. However, care recipients contribute to the caregiver's burnout, as well. Although no one chooses to become a care recipient, many do have control over their behavior. One client provided weeks of care after her twenty-three-year-old son underwent knee surgery. While the pain following his surgery was quite severe, in less than two weeks he managed to go back to work and resumed socializing with his friends. At home, however, he continued to whine and demand his mother's almost constant attention. Only when she began refusing his requests did he become more self-sufficient.

Another client reported that his emotionally troubled partner spent a small fortune on psychotherapy, but made no real effort to follow through on his therapist's recommendations. In cases like these, where the care recipient's response makes the caregiver's job more difficult, it's not surprising that resentments build.

No one likes being taken for granted or having their efforts to provide compassionate care go unappreciated. Yet, the care recipient may be struggling with too many conflicts to express gratitude. And, as noted earlier, many undergo personality changes, becoming sullen, demanding, even spiteful. In the case of dementia, the care recipient may be incapable of any coherent expression at all. In these cases, it is vital that caregivers find other sources of gratification, be especially vigilant about self-care, and be aware of their special risk for burnout.

Dealing with the Warning Signs of Burnout

"Okay," you say, "so I'm at risk for burnout. What can I do about it?" Regardless of which warning signs you are experiencing, there are steps you can take to cope with them when they appear.

Step One: *Name the feeling.* It's very upsetting to feel distressed without having a clear sense of what's going on. Identifying what you are feeling will help. For example, once you know that you are feeling pressured and overwhelmed (Item 3 in the inventory), you can start exploring ways to relieve the pressure. Similarly, once you realize that you are feeling isolated, you can work on reaching out to friends.

Step Two: *Identify the trigger.* Although they may seem to come from nowhere, feelings are always understandable reactions to thoughts or events. Think about what was going on just before the feeling appeared. Did your care recipient say something offensive or aggravating? Did you confront someone who has not been pitching in? Or perhaps you just thought of something you'd rather be doing.

Sometimes the trigger is easy to find. For example, one woman scolded her child when he asked for help with his math homework. "I knew I was overreacting," she said. "And I realized I must have been angry before Sean even asked me for help." When the woman thought about what had preceded her outburst, she recalled having been upset by her elderly father not five minutes previously, when he had criticized the "inedible" meal she had served him. She had wanted to say something, but the risk of upsetting the frail old man deterred her, so she tried, unsuccessfully, to shrug it off.

Sometimes, the trigger is not clear. In such cases, it's often helpful to ask yourself, "When have I felt like this before?" For example, one man felt upset, but could not identify the cause. When he began to focus on his body, he became aware of a hollow feeling in his stomach and a tightness in his throat. "As I felt these sensations," he recalled, "I thought about all those Saturday mornings as a kid when I had nothing to look forward to but chores and boredom!" At that moment he realized he was both angry and depressed, since he had nothing pleasant to anticipate for the entire day.

Step Three: *Accept your feelings.* Once you know what you are feeling, suspend judgment and accept the feeling as valid. You really have no choice—much as you might want to, you cannot wish it away. Once you can accept your feeling you can work toward a resolution.

Step Four: *Solve the problem.* Tempting though it might be, you really cannot tell your elderly father that he is an ungrateful lout. Nor should you phone your brother and yell at him for not helping you. Emotional outbursts are seldom helpful to anyone. Instead, focus on finding realistic solutions for your problems. In the next section of this chapter, we'll show you how to do this.

Coping Strategies

By the time a person is burnt out, the harm has already been done. Preventing this from happening requires awareness and discipline. On the following pages we offer suggestions to prevent burnout. The inventory that follows is based on the one you completed earlier in this chapter, but it encourages you to form an action plan to cope with the identified problem areas.

Preventing Burnout

Directions: Review your answers to the items in the inventory you completed earlier in the chapter (pp. 64–65). If you responded to an item affirmatively (by circling Y), carefully consider each set of questions that follows the statement below, then use the space provided to formulate your action plan. As you do so, be sure to consider exactly what you plan to do, when, and how.

We have completed the first item to give you an example:

1. I feel sad and "down" more often than is normal for me.   Y   N

   Questions to ask yourself: When do I feel better? Does anything cause my "down" mood to lift? For example, does a change in my daily routine help? Is my sadness related to anything I can control ? Do I get sad when I feel taken advantage of by others? If so, what can I do to help myself?

   My Plan: I will schedule a mid-morning "newspaper and coffee" break, starting tomorrow.

2. Lately, I am doing fewer of the things I enjoy.   Y   N

   Questions to ask yourself: Within the next few days, what would I enjoy doing? Is there a movie I'd like to see? A restaurant I want to try? A TV show I'd like to watch?

My Plan:

_____

_____

_____

3. I often feel overwhelmed and pressured. Y N

   Questions to ask yourself: Where is this pressure coming from? What can I do to reduce it? Can I delegate responsibilities? Accept offers of help from others? Reduce my other commitments?

   My Plan:

   _____

   _____

   _____

4. I feel very alone much of the time. Y N

   Questions to ask yourself: To whom might I talk? Can I call a friend? Is there someone, such as a rabbi or pastor, with whom I can share my distress?

   My Plan:

   _____

   _____

   _____

5. I often cry. Y N

   Questions to ask yourself: What words are my tears expressing? How can I help myself feel better?

   My Plan:

   _____

   _____

   _____

6. I prefer not to talk about my stresses or problems with others.
   Y   N

   Questions to ask yourself: Who might I feel safe talking with? How can I contact them? What lay or professional helpers are available to me?

   My Plan:

   _____

   _____

   _____

7. I sometimes feel my anger will get out of control.   Y   N

   Questions to ask yourself: When do I get angry? What can I do to direct that anger appropriately? Can I, for example, confront someone who is not doing his share?

   My Plan:

   _____

   _____

   _____

8. I react strongly to little annoyances.   Y   N

   Questions to ask yourself: Why am I reacting as I am? What do these strong reactions suggest? Where should my annoyance really be directed?

   My Plan:

   _____

   _____

   _____

9. I'm afraid I'll do something to injure my care recipient.   Y   N

   Questions to ask yourself: What am I angry about? Who can help me sort out my feelings? How can I come to grips with my anger and resentment? Could I benefit from speaking to a mental health specialist?

My Plan:

---

10. I resent it when other people have a good time. Y N

    Questions to ask yourself: What is causing me to feel this resentment? What positive steps can I take that would make my everyday life more pleasant?

    My Plan:

---

11. I feel "edgy" much of the time. Y N

    Questions to ask yourself: What is causing this "edgy" feeling? Am I giving myself time to unwind? Am I relying on caffeine or other substances to enable me to keep going when I really need to rest?

    My Plan:

---

12. I often feel something terrible is about to happen. Y N

    Questions to ask yourself: Since this is a symptom of anxiety, what steps can I take on my own to reduce my anxiety level? Could I benefit from a stress management group? Should I see a mental health profession to help me manage my anxiety?

    My Plan:

As you formulate your plans, please keep the following sources of information, guidance, and support in mind:

- Your personal physician or your care recipient's
- Your local hospital
- A nearby Visiting Nurses Association
- Local chapters of national organizations, such as the Alzheimer's Association (for information about community resources, including caregiver support groups)
- A senior center
- A family service agency in your area
- A local newspaper
- A local phone directory
- Books about stress management and stress reduction
- A research librarian

Additional information on taking care of yourself appears in chapter 5, "Self-Care for the Caregiver," where we offer specific suggestions about self-care. If any of your responses to the exercise on pages 70–73 indicate that you may be at risk for burnout, you might want to read that chapter now.

CHAPTER FIVE

SELF-CARE FOR THE CAREGIVER

In this chapter we explain why caregivers tend to ignore their own needs, and point out the dangers in doing so. We also stress the importance of being proactive with regard to self-care, and provide you with tools to assist you in this task.

The subject of self-care often elicits less than positive responses from caregivers. "Yeah, sure!" they say. "Just tell me when I'm supposed to make time for myself! I'm so busy, if I get to take a shower every day and talk with a friend on the phone I consider myself lucky! Exercise? Go to a museum? Spend a weekend with friends? Right!"

Chronically short of time, hounded by demands from all sides, they regard reminders to care for themselves as just another pressure to deal with. For example, one woman complained about being overweight and out of shape. A friend recommended that she join a gym and begin working out a few times a week. Since it seemed a logical thing to do, she agreed. Two weeks later it became apparent that accepting the advice had been a mistake. Because of the demands on her time, she'd been able to go only twice. She felt depressed, angry with herself, and guilty about having spent the money to join the gym.

Resistance to Self-Care

Listed below are the reasons caregivers typically give for avoiding self-care. Take a moment to read each of them, then formulate an argument to rebut it. At the end of this exercise, we'll add our arguments to yours.

Reason One: "It's not I who needs care! I'm the healthy one!"

Your Rebuttal: _____

_____

_____

_____

Reason Two: "It's selfish. I can't do that to my care recipient."

Your Rebuttal: _____

_____

_____

_____

Reason Three: "Others will think I'm irresponsible."

Your Rebuttal: _____

_____

_____

_____

Reason Four: "I'd never forgive myself if something happened while I was out having a good time!"

Your Rebuttal: _____

_____

_____

_____

Reason Five: "I shouldn't need to take a break. I'm strong."

Your Rebuttal:

_____

_____

_____

Now, compare our responses with yours.

Reason One: "It's not I who needs care! I'm the healthy one!"

We say: You won't be healthy for long if you don't take care of yourself. Overstressed caregivers are more likely to become ill, and their illnesses are likely to last longer. Self-care is a basic human right which you don't forfeit simply because you've become a caregiver. Workers take coffee breaks and vacations. Even prisoners are allowed to exercise and have visitors. By taking care of yourself, you are letting everyone know that you are a person, not a need-fulfilling object. Later in this chapter you'll learn how to avoid exploitation by establishing clear limits and boundaries.

Reason Two: "It's selfish. I can't do that to my care recipient."

We say: There is nothing selfish about taking care of your needs, and by taking care of yourself, you're more likely to take better care of your care recipient. In fact, by not taking care of yourself you may inadvertently be lapsing into the role of martyr. By being an anxious and overly solicitous caregiver, you do your care recipient no favor, and may hurt yourself in the process.

Reason Three: "Others will think I'm irresponsible."

We say: Nearly everyone has an opinion about almost everything, but the basis of these opinions is often highly personal. People who are inclined to judge others harshly typically lack objectivity, compassion, and detachment. Sometimes they are just plain self-righteous. To fear their judgment gives them power they don't deserve. Remember, only you know your needs, feelings, and stresses.

Reason Four: "I'd never forgive myself if something happened while I was out having a good time!"

We say: Some people, out of guilt, anticipate dire consequences if they do anything pleasurable. However, the reality is that when proper provision is made for someone to cover for you, the feared consequences rarely occur.

Reason Five: "I shouldn't need to take a break. I'm strong."

We say: That word *should* is dangerous and means you're at risk for ignoring how you actually feel. You may be depleted, angry, resentful, and frazzled, but if you are expecting yourself to be superwoman, you will feel obliged to push on. Recognize your limits and respect them.

The Importance of Being Proactive

The word proactive means taking an action before it's necessary. Being proactive as a caregiver means anticipating your own needs and seeking out opportunities to satisfy them, much as a physician tries to prevent illness by urging proper nutrition and a healthy lifestyle, or diligent parents "childproof" a home. It is unrealistic to expect others to know what your needs are, especially if you have a reputation for being strong. By being proactive, you are letting others know that you matter, and that you are entitled to take care of yourself.

Here's a mnemonic device you can use. We call it the Caregiver's S-T-O-P Sign. Call it to mind any time you are overburdened and doing more than you can comfortably handle.

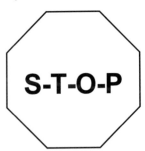

S: Seek out opportunities for support.

With a little effort, you can locate resources in your community. A caregiver group, for example, can provide both practical guidance and emotional support. Your local hospital or Area Agency on Aging, or a specialty group such as the Alzheimer's Association, will almost certainly be able to assist you.

T: Take time for the things you enjoy.

Although you may not have the time for an elaborate project, you can almost certainly find the time to do something you like. For example, instead of attending a concert, borrow a CD from your library. If you can't get to the movies, rent a video and make yourself some microwave popcorn. Avoid saying, "I can't do anything!" just because you can no longer do it the way you used to.

O: Opt for help whenever you can.

When someone offers to help, assume she means it and take her up on it. If you are inclined to say no automatically, learn to say yes. Should your care recipient protest, explain your plans, then follow through. Yielding invites tyranny; gentle firmness invites trust and respect.

P: Prioritize your needs.

Since you can't do everything you'd like to do, decide what's most important to you. If exercise matters more than meeting a friend for coffee, forget the coffee and get out your running shoes.

Here is a logsheet to provide an easy way to ensure you're taking care of yourself. Look at the sample page that follows, and read the examples. Duplicate page 80 to record what you've done, describe your feelings "before and after," and make a note of when you'll do the activity again. Use the "Remarks" column for any reminders that might be useful.

Caregiver's Logsheet					
Date	How I Felt Before	What I Did	How I Felt After	When Will I Do It Again?	Remarks
11/6/99	Depressed	Called Betty	Relieved	As necessary	Glad I reached out
11/7/99	Bored	Went for a walk	Refreshed	Daily, if possible	Need regular exercise

The following is for you to duplicate.

Caregiver's Logsheet

Date	How I Felt Before	What I Did	How I Felt After	When Will I Do It Again?	Remarks

Balancing Needs and Setting Boundaries

When you set boundaries, you clarify what you are willing to do. For example, "I'll pick you up after your appointment with the doctor. Ask the receptionist to call me ahead of time and let me know when you'll be done so I don't have to wait." Taking actions of this sort helps to reduce the frustration that comes from "wasting time."

The ease with which you can balance your own needs and those of your care recipient depends, in part, on the kind of caregiving responsibilities you have. In general, the more extensive and unremitting your care recipient's needs, the more difficult it is to keep things in check. If you have responsibilities to others (a partner, spouse, or children) you must factor those into your balancing act as well. A child's need for help with homework doesn't disappear when you become a caregiver. Your partner's need for companionship doesn't go away either.

If you work, you also have the demands of your job to consider. Even if everyone understands and is supportive of the accommodations you request, you must still fulfill your responsibilities. (This doesn't mean you should quit your job. Caregivers who do so almost always regret it. The regular contact with the "outside world" helps prevent a feeling of being trapped in the caregiving role.)

How to Set Boundaries

1. Delegate tasks to others. For each task to be accomplished, ask yourself: What needs to be done? Can it be divided up? Can anyone help with any of the parts?

Consider this example. Joan, a forty-one-year-old divorced caregiver with two teenage daughters, spent many months doing all the cleaning and cooking for herself, her children, and her elderly father. She was exhausted. When speaking to a friend one day she learned that her friend's daughters—who were the same ages as Joan's daughters—had begun preparing meals. Joan realized that her own youngsters could certainly take on at least some of the tasks of meal preparation. She talked the matter over with them and asked the two of them to make dinner at least twice a week. Each daughter took sole responsibility for one meal, and agreed to jointly prepare a third.

2. Have your care recipient take on as much responsibility as possible. In chapter 2 we mentioned that it's unwise to foster dependency. To avoid doing so, observe your own behavior

with these two questions in mind: (1) Is it necessary that I do this? and (2) Can my care recipient accomplish any part of this task without my help? An answer of "no" to the first question and "yes" to the second says that you are taking on unnecessary work.

3. Be willing to change your mind. If you take on a job and realize later that you really can't manage, speak up. One working woman volunteered to run errands and do the shopping for her ill neighbor, thereby sacrificing the little time she had to herself in the evening and on weekends. Once she realized the neighbor's son could do this, she shifted the responsibility to him. Similarly, if you say "no" to an invitation, and you then realize you made an error, call back and say "yes."

4. Identify the times of the day when problems consistently occur, then move some tasks to other time slots or get extra help. One man, for example, who was providing care for his seriously depressed wife, found that evenings were particularly difficult. At the end of the day, his wife was emotionally exhausted. She was refusing to eat or to take her medications. Shifting these activities to an earlier time of day reduced the chronic evening friction.

5. Re-evaluate problematic tasks; look for other ways of reaching the same goals. Sometimes an activity once needed is no longer necessary. In the weeks following her husband Jack's auto accident, Cynthia drove him to the gym for rehabilitation as soon as she got home from work. While he exercised, she cooked dinner and then drove back to pick him up—an extraordinarily inconvenient arrangement for her. She lived with this routine because Jack needed to use the specialized equipment available only at the gym. Even after his condition improved, the routine continued out of habit. Finally, one night, Cynthia blew up and accused Jack of taking her for granted. After she calmed down enough to discuss the problem, they met with Jack's physical therapist and arranged to rent one piece of exercise equipment. Jack's other exercises were re-formulated so they could be done at home. Jack's gain in autonomy and Cynthia's reduction in stress were a large payoff for relatively little effort.

In each of these instances, the caregiver took stock of the situation and made changes to reduce her stress and fatigue. And everyone benefited from the caregivers' actions.

CHAPTER SIX

HOW TO GET HELP WHEN OTHERS AREN'T HELPFUL

In this chapter, we offer suggestions on how to solve the problems most often faced by caregivers. We propose ways of fostering family cooperation, solving problems in the workplace, getting the best out of health-care providers, and protecting your interests when dealing with insurance company employees.

Geraldine got the call from the nursing home admissions officer on Thursday. A bed had become available, and her mother could be admitted the following Monday. This was much earlier than anyone had predicted. There was only one catch. Josephine's Medicaid application was incomplete. For her to be admitted, the home required, by Monday morning, a complete set of checking account statements dating back three years. "I don't have that stuff!" Geraldine blurted. She was shocked and dismayed at the request. "My mother throws out her bank statements. Half the time, she doesn't even understand them!" "I'm sorry, Mrs. Greene," the woman said, impersonally. "We can't do anything unless we have that information. If you can't get it to us by Monday, your mother's bed will be given to the next person on the list. And we can't predict when another bed will become available." "But," Geraldine began, "today is already Thursday. . . ." "I'm sorry." The woman was curt now. "I have another call coming in. What would you like to do?" Geraldine paused. "I'll get the information," she answered, not quite believing herself as she said the words. "Very good!" said the victorious woman, sourly and without interest. When Geraldine heard the click on the line, she muttered, "Bitch."

The next two days were a nightmare. Early Friday morning, she called her mother's bank. Geraldine inhaled, preparing to request help brightly and calmly, not wanting to betray the urgency she felt. "We're sorry," said the recorded voice on the phone. "All of our representatives are busy serving other customers. Your call will be answered in the order it was received." And then, "Thank you for your patience. Your call is very important to us. Someone will be with you in just a moment. "Geraldine, annoyed by phone messages conveying false concern, did not feel reassured. One minute later, she heard the same message. And again, a minute later. Finally a person answered.

Geraldine started to explain the situation. She had hardly begun when the person interrupted. "One moment!" Then the line went dead. There was a click. "We're sorry," the voice began again, "all of our representatives . . ." After the recorded announcement, there was another two-minute wait. Finally someone answered. "Mr. Wenick," said a new voice. "May I help you?" Geraldine wanted to ask why the first person had been so rude as to leave the line after only a few seconds without any explanation. But she thought better of it. "Yes, Mr. Wenick," she began. "My mother, Josephine Gennaro, has had a checking account with your bank for many years . . . ." She told him the story and the reason for her call. Mr. Wenick paused after she'd finished. "I'm sorry," he said. "The bank can't release records in response to a phone call. You'll need to come in to the bank in person. And you'll need—uh, let's see . . ." He paused, obviously reading something. "We'll need an authorization form," he began again, "signed by your mother and notarized."

And so it went. Geraldine's explanations and entreaties were useless. Eventually, she asked to be transferred to a supervisor, then a customer relations officer. Three hours and four phone calls later, the bank finally compromised. Someone would fax the authorization form to Geraldine. She would have it signed and notarized (a notary was willing to come to her home to witness her mother's signature for the exorbitant fee of $125), and fax it back to them. As soon as the bank got it, they would arrange to send the records to the nursing home. By one P.M., she had received the authorization form on her fax machine. That was the way Geraldine's entire day went. Like so many caregivers, she found that every time she tried to accomplish a task, she encountered people who were either rude, uncaring, or inflexible.

What do you do when you encounter such situations? How do you get help from individuals and institutions who aren't cooperative? We've identified three main areas of difficulty, and on the following pages, we discuss the planning and negotiation skills essential for coping with each. First, we'll talk about managing difficulties that arise within your family, when siblings don't do their share, or when your partner or children refuse to cooperate. Next, we'll discuss problems in the workplace, a common trouble spot for many caregivers. We'll also propose ways of handling nonresponsiveness on the part of the medical establishment, including health-care professionals and insurance company and HMO employees.

Solving Problems That Originate in the Family

In this section, we will offer advice on how to secure the cooperation of your siblings, as well as your spouse and children.

Why Siblings Won't Help

The typical family caregiver receives little or no help from other family members. There is no simple explanation for this, but when a group of family members (who had been described as "not helpful" by their caregiving siblings) were surveyed, they offered the following explanations. Their comments are typical.

- "I do plenty," said one man whose sister cared for their two elderly parents, "and I resent being made to feel I don't do enough! No matter what my sister says about how much she needs my help, the truth is she wants to run the show. She says she wants help, but every time I offer to help, it's the wrong time."

- A woman whose brother was being cared for by their mother said, "Yes, I could do more to help Mom take care of Fred, but I don't want to—especially since she always liked him better than me anyway."

- Another woman, a college professor, observed, "I have no patience with sick people. I'm just not cut out to be a caregiver."

- Other responses were much less gracious. One man said, "I don't have any time, interest, or desire. And who are you to be asking me this?"

The comments of the first man reveal his resentment at having had his offers of help rejected. Assuming that his offers were indeed timely, it appears that his sister unconsciously sought to exclude him from direct caregiving responsibilities, while simultaneously fostering guilt. Both siblings ended up feeling angry and resentful, without any awareness of what was going on.

In the second case, this respondent's unwillingness to help her mother was clearly tied to her anger at having felt "second-best" in relation to her brother.

The college professor would have to confront her discomfort with sick people before she could meaningfully offer help.

The anger of the last man probably covers up a welter of feelings that he would rather not face. Such reactions are not unusual among people who have been identified as "not helpful" by caregivers. They feel threatened when asked about their lack of involvement. As unpleasant as their responses may seem, their refusal to answer in any depth may indicate discomfort rather than lack of caring.

Why Your Current Family Won't Cooperate

In a 1997 survey, the National Family Caregivers Association (1998) asked caregivers where they provide care. Eighty percent reported that their recipient lives with them. In such cases, all family members must accommodate to the presence of the care recipient. For example, when grandma moves in, a child may be asked to give up his bedroom and share a sibling's room. Often, children must learn to fend for themselves—cook their own dinner, for example—because the caregiver no longer has the time. One little girl complained that while she loved her grandmother, she hated having to be quiet all the time, and she hated not being able to have "sleepovers." "Grandma is sick," she pouted. "Not me!"

As this comment suggests, the presence of the care recipient may dominate family life, causing considerable distress to other family members. For example, a boy with attention deficit disorder (ADD) so dictated life at home that his entire family became caregivers. An older sister ensured that he took his medication. A younger one picked up after him. Everyone became quite expert at anticipating his impulsive behavior. Most family activities were planned with him in mind.

The members of the caregiver's current family inevitably vary in their willingness to help and in their ability to do so. One man, for example, simply assumed that his wife would be able to manage the responsibilities of homemaking, child care, and a part-time job, while caring for her elderly mother. Not until his wife became physically ill did he realize she needed assistance.

Other partners may avoid helping because of negative associations from their own past. Sheryl and Connie are an excellent case in point. As an adolescent, Sheryl had watched her mother slowly die of cancer. Her grief, coupled with the sights, sounds, and smells of sickness, remained deeply etched in her memory. When her partner's mother was diagnosed with cancer, Sheryl spoke candidly to Connie. "I can't do this!" she confessed. "I wish I could." Her memories were too painful. Hence, her support for Connie was limited to her taking on most of the household responsibilities so that her partner would be free to care for her mother.

Sometimes the age of family members is a factor. For a short time after her mother's hospitalization, Juana's children rallied to her side. But the girls, being adolescents, were very much involved in their own lives. After the initial novelty of visiting grandma in the hospital wore off, they lost interest and seldom did anything to make their mother's life any easier.

Family history may also play a part in the extent to which family members give assistance. A man with a history of strained relationships with his in-laws can hardly be expected to throw himself into helping them when they grow old. Similarly, two brothers who have never gotten along with each other aren't likely to become close under the strain of caring for an aging parent.

When the lack of cooperation on the part of family members is the result of simple miscommunication, a direct statement of needs and concerns may be all that is needed. But when it stems from long-standing difficulties that may have little to do with caregiving issues, the assistance of a skilled and neutral mediator may be necessary. If you are not sure which situation applies to your family, we would suggest that as long as everyone seems willing to get together and talk, you should give that a try. The following section provides explicit guidelines for that process.

How to Obtain Cooperation from Your Family

To elicit more cooperation from your family, you must do four things: (1) acknowledge the existence of a problem, (2) talk about how it came about and what might be done to solve it, (3) create a plan for solving it, and (4) periodically evaluate your family's progress once the solution is implemented.

1. Acknowledge the Existence of the Problem

Many families are reluctant to admit that a problem exists. We noted earlier that struggles over caregiving often reflect much deeper difficulties. To illustrate, we'd like to tell the story of an actual client. Mr. K had had a variety of minor illnesses—upper respiratory infections, back problems, and headaches—for many months. When asked about how he became a caregiver, he said that he was the youngest of three children. He was a childless widower when his mother became ill at age eighty-five, and he took on all the caregiving responsibilities for her. For the next four years he struggled alone to meet her needs, never complaining. When asked how he felt about his siblings' lack of involvement, he responded without obvious bitterness. "As far as my family goes, there's really no problem. I can do this, so there's no reason why I shouldn't. I can't complain about my sister. She's so stressed with her career that I just can't ask her to do more. And my older brother has a family, so he can't do much either."

Before Mr. K could begin to redistribute responsibilities more fairly with his two siblings, he needed to realize that a problem even existed.

2. Talk About the Problem

Mr. K was persuaded to ask both his brother and his sister to meet with him to discuss their mother's care arrangements. The meeting was to take place with one of the authors present to facilitate. To move the process along, Mr. K was given a set of planning guidelines. He, in turn, sent a copy of the guidelines to each of his siblings.

Here are those guidelines, stated in a general form so that you can adapt them to your particular situation:

State your personal agenda. Before the meeting, each person attending should write down a few key concerns, and set priorities for each. If one person has initiated the meeting, then she should be especially clear about why she wants to meet. In the case of Mr. K, the issue was the uneven distribution of caregiving duties. In other cases, the topics might be expenses, nursing home decisions, or plans for the future.

Gather the facts. Someone, usually the initiator, should bring copies of all key information to the meeting to distribute to everyone. The information should include: (a) data about the care recipient, including history of the illness, current condition, diagnosis and prognosis, and medications; (b) information about the responsibilities assumed by the caregiver (kinds of services provided, amount of time spent daily or weekly providing care); and (c) any other factors that warrant a review of existing care arrangements, such as changes in the care recipient's condition. In the case in question, Mr. K wrote a few paragraphs about the allocation of family responsibilities, and identified changes he wanted to see.

Set goals. Everyone present should agree on the outcomes that will indicate that the meeting has succeeded. To Mr. K, "success" meant that both his brother and sister would take on some of the caregiving responsibilities. It also meant he would be able to schedule a two-week vacation for himself, something he hadn't done in four years. The goal of the meeting should be stated clearly and without equivocation. For example, in the case of the K family, the problem was clearly stated in this manner: "We're here to talk about how the burdens of caring for Mom can be more evenly distributed among all of us." This is preferable to a more imprecise goal such as, "We're here to discuss how Mom can be cared for better."

Set communication guidelines. During the meeting, the following three rules of communication may prove helpful, especially when there is likely to be conflict.

- First, family members should listen to one another, without interrupting, in order to understand each other's perspectives. (If the family is large, or if some people tend to interrupt or to talk incessantly, it may be necessary to set time limits.) Before responding to each other's comments, people can be asked to restate each other's messages in their own words, just to ensure understanding before any response is made.

- Second, people should speak only for themselves and not for anyone else. They should use "I messages" rather than "you messages" and avoid preaching, judging, blaming, and giving advice.

- Third, any communication between members of the family should be public. To ensure the success of the meeting, there must be no silent agreements or secret exchanges.

3. **Create a Plan for Solving the Problem**

The key outcome of the meeting should be a plan for a solution to the problems that have been identified. In the case of the K family, the plan involved fair allocation of responsibilities. The family members agreed that care should be provided not only by them-selves, but also by people from the community, including visiting nurses, home-health aides, and companions.

You may find the following steps helpful in creating a plan:

- **Air feelings.** Before any rational problem solving can take place, if strong emotions are involved, they must be vented. All family members should be given a chance to air their grievances, voice their concerns, and unburden themselves.

- **Clarify.** To make the issues clear to everyone, the origins and effects of the problem should be spelled out. This requires answering these questions:

  - What should be happening now that isn't?

  - What is happening now that shouldn't be?

  - Why does the problem exist?

  - What will happen if we do nothing?

- **Gather and review data.** All the pertinent facts should be assembled and reviewed. This includes data about the care recipient's diagnosis, prognosis, medications, nature and extent of care required, and expenses. It also includes other pertinent information such as professional and community resources. In the case of the K family, since the homework required was substantial, it was necessary to schedule three family meetings to allow time for data gathering and discussion. This is not at all unusual.

- **Propose solutions.** At this point, family members brainstorm to generate possible solutions. By thinking ahead, family members can identify potential problems. After all the facts were gathered, the members of the K family began dividing up what needed to be done and by whom. Each proposal was evaluated for practicality, workability, and effective-ness. They talked about holidays, summer vacations, and so on. The plan they came up with included arrangements for both routine care and atypical situations. The plan was well thought-out and allowed for flexibility in case of special cir-cumstances.

4. Periodically Evaluate Progress

It's wise to plan to meet periodically to review the outcomes of your problem solving. Is the plan working? Has the problem been solved? If not, why not? Is fine-tuning required? All family problem solving follows these steps in one way or another. Regardless of the type of problem, this procedure, when used by people acting in good faith, will almost always result in a solution.

Mental Illness in a Caregiving Team Member

Occasionally, the caregiving situation is complicated by the presence of a family member with a significant mental illness, whose inappropriate behaviors may antagonize other family members and outside professionals. Consider these words, written by one of three siblings responsible for the care of an elderly mother. The writer, a woman, lives many hundreds of miles from her mother and siblings.

"So much of my experience as a caregiver is colored by the fact that my brother, Abe, is mentally ill. Lynn and I work together well and basically what I have done is to be available (via phone and email) as a source of moral support, a sounding board, and joint decision maker for her. I just got a desperate call from her last night that Abe had been in overdrive mode again, browbeating her and telling her that if she doesn't do more, I'll have to come back again. Lynn told Abe that that was out of the question.

"Trying to do reality checking with Abe is very draining. Despite the fact that he complains constantly about our mother not having met his needs as a child, he needs to feel that he is the only one who is really working hard to help Mom now. Lynn and I don't buy into Abe's guilt tripping because we know we are doing everything we can. We keep trying to explain to Abe that even if all three of us were available to work full-time on providing for our mother's care, it still would not be enough. We have to accept the fact that, despite our best efforts, the care is not yet adequate.

"In the meantime, Lynn has found a nursing home and is waiting for a bed to become available. She is working out a lot of financial matters with yet another elder-law attorney. Abe leaves messages on Lynn's answering machine demanding that she call back late at night, which involves listening to Abe's monologues. Lynn has been doing extraordinary work and has been very mindful of Abe's feelings. Anyone would be exhausted and have some emotional conflicts under the never-ending strain of this situation, but Abe's paranoia and other inappropriate behaviors really add to our burden."

To cope with situations like this, it is essential that intact family members acknowledge the mental illness. In some families, there is such a stigma associated with this that even flagrantly bizarre behaviors may be dismissed as merely "odd." Once the existence of mental illness has been accepted, the next step is to determine whether the affected family member can participate in family decisions without being unduly disruptive. Even when her participation will not be helpful, if it matters to her to be present, she may need to be included. If her presence would be disruptive, and she can be excluded, that is what should be done. If excluding her creates conflict among the other caregivers, it may be advisable to enlist the aid of a professional who has expertise in dealing with mental illness, and is comfortable actively setting limits. The disturbed individual cannot be allowed to disrupt or sabotage the efforts of other family members.

Solving Problems in the Workplace

According to Sue Shellenbarger of *The Wall Street Journal* (1997), 50 percent of employed caregivers reported that they had missed work time because of caregiving responsibilities.

Some employers have liberal policies that allow job sharing (two or more people cooperate to fulfill the responsibilities of one job); flex-time (employees arrive at work earlier or later than normal, leave during the day if necessary, and end the workday earlier or later); and other accommodations. Nevertheless, too many employers remain unsympathetic to the needs of caregivers. Melanie, a young widow with two special needs teens, struggled for two years to satisfy her employer while taking her children to appointments and picking them up from after-school tutoring. Eventually she found it necessary to quit her job because she was unable to do her work adequately. Employers such as hers are shortsighted, adhering to policies that result in the loss of good employees.

What to Do About Workplace Problems

Many workplace arrangements are made informally, as, for example, when a responsible employee approaches a reasonable superior and explains that caregiving responsibilities require that she leave early on a given day. Similarly, flex-time and job-sharing arrangements can often be negotiated among co-workers. As long as an employee doesn't abuse the good faith of superiors and colleagues, and as long as company policies are flexible and reasonable, these arrangements can work. However, informal arrangements are not always possible. In such cases, you need to know what your legal rights are.

On February 5, 1993, President Bill Clinton signed into law the federal Family and Medical Leave Act, which took effect on August 5th of that year. Touted as a breakthrough in United States official family policy, the Act guarantees twelve weeks of unpaid leave annually for every employee in the United States in order to provide care for a family member and for other reasons (e.g., maternity leave). The law specifies that the leave may be taken in one block or a few days at a time. Regardless of how the time is used, the employer must continue to pay for the employee's health insurance and other benefits during the leave period. Moreover, the employee is guaranteed his or her job back.

Unfortunately, according to *The Wall Street Journal* (Schellenbarger 1994), not all employers are making a concerted effort to implement the law. Many are not informing employees of their rights and training supervisors to implement the law. Nevertheless, you do have the right to take advantage of its provisions.

Although you have the right to the family leave, your request should be made with full awareness of your employer's and co-workers' needs. Here are various situations you may encounter, and ways of managing them.

How to Request Concessions

1. Be sensitive to your employer's needs.

When requesting concessions, be sure to follow the proper chain of command and try to minimize the disruption created by your request. Remember, your boss has a job to do; he or she is not a social worker.

As always, we urge you to use good communication techniques. Avoid "you should" messages that are blaming and judgmental. Instead, express your feelings and needs by means of "I messages." For example, "I really appreciate your understanding in this situation. My mother's illness is not something I welcome, but I'm the only child who can care for her now."

2. Be clear about your goals, but strive for a "win-win" outcome.

In his masterful little book, *You Can Negotiate Anything* (1989), Herb Cohen speaks about a variety of negotiation styles. Some people are intent on winning at all costs. They care little about the feelings or needs of the other party or about maintaining goodwill, and so they frequently end up creating ill will and undermining relationships. Any victory is, therefore, a hollow one, since the "loser" will almost certainly be upset.

By contrast, a "win-win" negotiation is a process designed to help both sides meet their needs. It is characterized by candor and cooperation, the very opposite of the heavy-handed approach just described. Everyone involved can come away from the encounter feeling satisfied that they were treated fairly.

3. **Make it easy for your superiors to give you what you want.**

Before approaching your superiors, speak with co-workers and try to elicit their cooperation. In that way you can reassure your boss that others are prepared to pick up any slack resulting from accommodations made on your behalf. Also, consider offering to fulfill some of your job responsibilities from home. One client moved several hundred miles away from his workplace for a few months, but was able to use a computer and modem to continue doing his job well.

The Period of Leave

Your task is not completed once your leave is granted. There are certain courtesies you should extend during this period.

1. Keep your employer informed about how things are going. Has your situation changed? Will these changes affect your anticipated date of return?

2. Demonstrate your responsibility by asking to be brought up-to-date from time to time. Call, or use email or fax. Even better, if possible, stop in at the office and ask to be updated.

After the Leave Ends

Once your leave has ended, be sure to express appreciation to everyone who has accommodated you. Do whatever you can to ease your transition back to your normal schedule. For example, if you did a substantial amount of independent work, prepare a summary for your superiors and co-workers.

Solving Problems with Health-Care Professionals

Caregiving involves considerable stress. Compassionate treatment by medical professionals can help a great deal. Unfortunately, it is not typical. Gary Barg, editor of the magazine, *Today's Caregiver*, identified several qualities you and your care recipient have the right to expect from a health-care provider. They are the following:

1. **Attentiveness.** Your recipient may be the fifth patient with dementia seen by his physician today, but to you this person is Mom or Dad. Medical personnel need to be as attentive as if your recipient were their only patient.

2. **Compassion, understanding, and empathy.** Your feelings, and those of your recipient, deserve to be taken seriously. Insensitivity, whether due to fatigue, overwork, or poor office practices is not something to which you or your care recipient should be subjected. Too many health-care providers lack empathy, as in the case of the physician who chided a woman for crying upon learning that her cancer had reappeared.

3. **Time.** Your health-care professional can give considerable support by providing a few moments of undivided attention. One physician we know plans her workday to allow plenty of time to speak with patients and their caregivers, believing she can learn a great deal about how to help her patients by doing so. Not surprisingly, her compassionate attitude has gained her appreciation from patients and a steady flow of referrals from peers.

4. **Respect.** Health-care providers demonstrate respect by making an effort to learn names and by taking questions and concerns seriously. They show respect when they explain what they are doing. And they show respect when they take the time to tell patients and their caregivers what to expect when tests or other procedures are recommended. Here are some examples of the kind of information that should be provided:

   • What exactly will the care recipient experience when he undergoes this test?

   • Are there any special discomforts associated with this procedure?

   • How long will the procedure take?

   Health-care providers show respect in still other ways. When a number of treatment options exist, for example, they help you decide among them. They also make appropriate referrals when the limits of their knowledge or experience have been exceeded.

5. **Dedication.** The best providers are willing to go the extra mile for you and your charge. That may mean making a phone call at the end of the workday to ask how your care recipient is doing, or to ask how he is tolerating a new medication. It may mean calling a physical therapist on the patient's behalf to ensure that proper treatment is provided.

6. **Candor.** Competent providers give needed information in a straightforward manner. In one case, for example, a physician took the time to explain to a patient that the medication he was prescribing would likely cause some mild stomach distress for a day or two, but assured him that the benefits were worth the inconvenience. In another, a physician gave her patient three treatment options, then carefully explained why one option was clearly preferable to the other two.

7. **Willingness to advocate.** During these times of managed care and Hospital Utilization Review Boards, patients often depend on a physician's willingness to "make waves" to see that they get proper care. In one case, for example, a doctor learned that his patient's managed care company had refused to authorize needed psychotherapy. He immediately called the case manager and persuaded her to grant the authorization. Unfortunately, many physicians are unwilling to extend themselves. For example, one hospital psychiatrist refused to contest his Utilization Review Board's recommendation that a severely depressed client be discharged. She was sent home after only a few days in the hospital, despite the family's protests. The very next day she attempted suicide, resulting in a lawsuit against both the doctor and the hospital.

8. **Willingness to educate patients and their families.** Family caregivers consistently identify this as essential. Too few physicians provide needed information and instruction, a situation with increasingly serious implications. In a June 1998 article in *The New York Times*, Ian Fisher reported that in an effort to reduce health-care costs, family caregivers are increasingly asked to perform highly technical procedures at home, often without receiving adequate training and preparation. Highly sophisticated equipment, intimidating to use, has made it possible for them to provide care once administered only by physicians and nurses. Unfortunately, medical personnel often don't take the time required to familiarize family caregivers with these machines. One sixty-five-year-

old woman, whom Fisher interviewed, reported that a nurse had spent only five minutes teaching her to use the complex piece of computerized equipment required to monitor her husband's condition after his discharge from the hospital. Such insensitivity not only adds to the stress of family caregiving, but may increase the likelihood of medical complications.

What to Do

To get the responses you want from medical and health personnel, we recommend that you follow these three steps:

1. **Be clear about your needs.** Do you need education? Information? A review of treatment alternatives and their consequences? Do you need to have terms explained? Procedures written down?

Do not be afraid to ask for what you need. Don't be satisfied with responses that give little real information. Ask all the questions you need to and don't stop until you understand the answers.

2. **Insist that your rights be respected.** If ever you are concerned that any right has been (or even could be) violated, express that concern as soon as the threat becomes apparent.

3. **If you are dissatisfied, tell your health-care provider.** Rather than complaining elsewhere or finding another doctor, speak with the professional involved. Physicians and other health-care providers aren't mind readers. When verbalizing your complaint, follow these guidelines:

- Be specific. State exactly what happened, when, and why you are dissatisfied. For example, "Doctor Abrams, last Thursday, during our eleven A.M. meeting, you said you would arrange to have a prescription called in to my local pharmacy later that day. I checked with the drugstore three hours later, and no call had been made. I phoned your office immediately and was told by your nurse that she had no record of your having asked her to phone in a prescription for me. She said she would double-check with you and call me right back. Twenty-four hours passed, and I received no call. When I called the pharmacy again, they told me that they had never heard from your office." This kind of complaint is neither a whine nor a demand, but a reasonable, believable, and documented account of a problem.

- Follow up with a letter. Regardless of whether the matter is cleared up to your satisfaction, a brief letter reviewing what occurred will remind the doctor of the problem, and provide motivation to see that the same kind of thing doesn't happen again. If thanks are in order, your letter can include those as well.

Simple candor is often enough to resolve problems with physicians and other health-care providers. Talk. Address problems quickly. Think of yourself as a partner in the treatment. Do all you can to prevent minor problems from escalating into major ones. Spare yourself the trouble of finding a new provider, as well as the unpleasantness, cost, and emotional trauma of a lawsuit.

Solving Problems with Insurance Company Employees

Ian Fisher, whose article we referred to earlier, notes that in this age of managed care, the pressures to reduce health-care costs are enormous. Far too often, the goal of the case manager and other employees of managed care organizations is to find a reason to deny benefits. Consider these instances:

- The brain-injured physician about whom we wrote earlier remained seriously impaired three years after his accident. He was clearly unable to process information rapidly and accurately, or to express himself adequately. Yet when he saw an IME (an "independent" medical examiner, who was, in reality, a pawn of the insurance company) this physician insisted the patient was able to return to work! "Yeah!" he said "And I'd like the IME to be my first patient!"

- A single parent, whose older daughter had undergone serious knee surgery, had a similar experience. Although at one time the surgical procedure would have required several nights' stay at the hospital, it has become a one-day affair, with rehabilitation provided on an out-patient basis. In this case, the youngster was on a variety of medications and needed to have her blood levels checked periodically. On the planned day of discharge, neither the woman nor her daughter were given any instructions on follow-up care. No arrangements were made for checking her blood levels or for physical therapy; it was simply assumed that her mother, who worked full-time and had limited financial resources, would figure out what to do by herself.

Dealing with Your Care Recipient's Insurance Company

Managed care companies, including HMOs (Health Maintenance Organizations) and PPOs (Preferred Provider Organizations) have earned the reputation of failing to respond to the needs of the people they serve. Some limit care inappropriately and refuse to authorize payment for reasonable and necessary medical procedures.

Unfortunately, at the present time, you must be prepared for the possibility that your care recipient may be victimized in this way. You need to know how to contest denial of services and how to persuade others to advocate on your charge's behalf.

Managed care companies abuse their power in three ways: (1) They may deny authorization for a service or procedure outright. (2) They may authorize a service, and then withdraw their approval. (Sometimes, after the procedure has been performed, the doctor is simply not paid. At that point he or she may turn to you for payment.) (3) Finally, the companies may deny payment of a claim for a service on some technicality. Often, such denials are described as "nonnegotiable" and "final." Intimidation is definitely a factor here. These companies know that few customers will challenge their decision. They count on fear, ignorance, and your lack of time.

What, then, can you do to advocate on behalf of your health-care recipient? The following recommendations are based on our own experience as health-care providers and as caregivers, supplemented by the expert, published recommendations of two attorneys familiar with the tactics routinely used by HMOs. Keep the following three principles in mind.

- First, do not assume that the HMO representative necessarily cares about your concerns or those of your care recipient.

- Second, do not count on cooperation in your efforts to seek fairness and adequate care. Prepare for the possibility that the relationship will become adversarial.

- Finally, remember that if you do not aggressively look after the interests of your care recipient, no one else will. The responsibility rests with you.

With those premises in mind, this is what you can do. Particulars will vary from one situation to the next and will depend on whether a request for authorization is denied before a service is performed, or whether a service previously authorized has not been paid for.

1. **Know your rights.** You must become familiar with the terms of your insurance contract. If you are unclear about any of your rights, or if the contract is difficult to understand, get help from your company's benefits officer, a more experienced caregiver, or even an attorney.

2. **Persist in calling and writing.** If the recommended service or procedure is something that should be covered, insist on it. If it is denied, ask for a written statement of the reasons for the denial. Get the names and credentials of the people involved in the decision. (If the decision involves a medical specialty, then a specialist in that area should be a part of the decision-making panel.)

3. **Ask your benefits officer or human resources administrator for help.** Let them know you are dissatisfied and why. Show your physician's written statement of need to your benefits officer. If you have been treated rudely by the HMO personnel, document your claim with names, dates, length or time kept waiting, and all other pertinent details.

4. **Save all documents, including bills and letters.** Date all correspondence you received and organize it neatly, using the logsheets provided on pages 101–102.

5. **Put as much information in writing as possible.** Send important letters by registered mail, return receipt requested, and keep copies of everything. Keep accurate phone records. Note the date and times of your calls. Document "wait time" and "disconnections," if any. If you were promised return calls but never received them, make a note of that, too. Always get the full name of each person with whom you speak. Record this information on a phone log sheet. (See sample log sheets on pages 103–104.)

6. **Turn to your physician's office personnel for help.** Many are insurance specialists. They can often supply information required to justify payment or to document the need for a service or procedure. They can guide you, and may even be willing to share their knowledge of specific people to ask for when you call the HMO.

Log Sheet: Letters Received

Date	Item Received	From Whom	Content of Message	Other

Log Sheet: Letters Sent

Date	Item Sent	To Whom	Content of Message	Other

Log Sheet: Telephone Calls Received

Date	Who Called	Caller's Number	Content of Message	Other

Date	Person Called	Their Number	Content of Message	Other

Log Sheet: Telephone Calls Placed

7. **Use your physician's written justification for the recommended service or procedure to make your case as persuasive as possible.**

8. **If necessary, file a complaint with your state's insurance commissioner.** Over the past several years, many abuses on the part of managed care companies have come to light. As a result, most states have begun passing legislation that provides protection for consumers. By describing your complaint and documenting it, you will almost certainly secure assistance.

9. **As a last resort, file a claim in small claims court or hire a lawyer.** These courses of action are time-consuming and may be expensive. However, we urge you to do all you can to force the insurer to honor the contract.

For years, too many managed care companies have been exploiting patients and growing wealthy on the pain and suffering of others. If you follow our recommendations aggressively and consistently, you will have a good chance of having your care recipient receive all the care and services to which he is entitled.

CHAPTER SEVEN

HIDDEN CAREGIVERS

In this chapter you will learn about a group of caregivers who don't think of themselves as such. Hidden caregivers routinely perform tasks for others who, in fact, are perfectly capable of taking care of themselves and who ought to be doing so. The term refers primarily to spouses who provide for needy and dependent partners, and children who feel responsible for meeting emotional and social needs of dysfunctional parents.

In the typical caregiving situation, there is a clearly identified caregiver, an easily recognizable care recipient, and an illness or disability that can be observed and acknowledged readily. Sometimes, however, the situation is not so clear. Although a relationship may appear to be normal, when it is looked at closely, what emerges is a dysfunctional pattern, in which one individual does more than her share in response to the other person's inability to fulfill everyday responsibilities.

Are You a Hidden Caregiver?

Hidden caregivers are people who have taken on a caregiving role without realizing they have done so. They don't think of themselves as caregivers and they don't realize that the help they give is, in reality, caregiving. They provide care for individuals who have not been identified as having an illness, addiction, or disability, and who often appear to be functioning quite normally. The recipients generally behave in an appropriate manner and have few obvious lapses.

Furthermore, their often incessant requests may be small, innocuous, and apparently reasonable. Because many of their ways of behaving are, in a mild form, considered normal, it's often difficult to recognize when the line has been crossed and real emotional dysfunction exists. Consider these examples:

- A husband who cannot decide what to wear to work or to a social function without help

- A mother who relies exclusively on her children for emotional support and companionship

- A friend who calls several times a day to seek guidance and reassurance on everything from work problems to child-rearing

- A homemaker who cannot run errands by herself

- A wife who cannot amuse herself and requires constant companionship

How can you determine when needs are excessive and reflect a "hidden caregiving" situation? To gauge this, look at the frequency, intensity, duration, and consequences of the person's needs.

Frequency

How often are the person's needs expressed? Hidden care recipients are usually unrelenting in their demands. They have little awareness of the impact of their demands on others, and they seem never to be satisfied. For example, one man was incapable of preparing even the simplest of meals on his own. When his wife took a week's vacation, she felt obliged to prepare all his meals in advance—almost as though he were disabled.

In extreme cases, hidden care recipients may even lie and manipulate when they cannot get what they need more forthrightly.

Intensity

How urgently is the need expressed? Usually, hidden care recipients convey a sense of urgency about their needs. They may look crestfallen if they do not get what they want. A woman may cry. A man may become angry, cold, or withdrawn. One father was so dependent on his pre-teenage son for companionship that when the child declined his offer to go shopping, he behaved as though a personal injury had been inflicted on him.

Duration

Is the person always in need of care? On a short-term basis, anyone can be "down" and in need of help. But when this becomes a way of life—when an individual is always in need—he becomes a hidden care recipient.

Consequences

Another way of estimating whether a hidden caregiving situation exists is to examine the outcomes of the care recipient's neediness. Usually, hidden caregivers wind up frustrated, embroiled in impossible and absurd situations. They may take on their recipients' battles and assume extraordinary responsibility for their well-being. Caregivers of such people often wind up doing what they don't want to do and wondering how they ever got themselves into that situation.

Hidden Caregiving Is Insidious

What makes hidden caregiving so difficult to detect is the fact that the extraordinary demands of hidden care recipients only become apparent over time. The situation is truly insidious. Hidden care recipients do not realize what a drain they are on the people around them. Confronted with the idea that they are emotional sink-holes, they would likely be hurt and accuse their caregivers of being selfish and of overreacting. Hidden caregivers, usually unaware of what is happening, are typically confused about the source of their exhaustion and resentment.

An ironic twist may occur in these situations. If the unidentified care recipient actually becomes a legitimate care recipient, the already overburdened caregiver may resent this additional burden, and refuse to respond appropriately. For example, the wife of an unidentified care recipient felt chronically put-upon by her husband's never-ending neediness: "I can't find my keys!" "Where are the blue slacks that go with this shirt?" "I lost my glasses again, honey! Would you help me find them?" When this man underwent minor surgery, his wife refused to take care of him. Instead, she had his co-workers take him to the hospital and bring him home.

In another case, the husband of an anxious and needy woman looked after her endlessly, anticipating her moods and accompanying her to places to which she wouldn't travel alone. When she required a biopsy for possible breast cancer, her husband's rage emerged. Not only did he refuse to accompany her to the hospital, but he also refused, the following week, to go with her to obtain the results of the test. Instead, he went to work as usual, and received the results at the end of the day.

Unaware of the basis for their rage, these two hidden caregivers felt guilty and embarrassed by their behavior, and thought of themselves as cold and heartless. Only when they understood what had happened did they realize just how angry and resentful they were.

By its very nature, hidden caregiving may be difficult to differentiate from normally caring behaviors. The following exercise can help you to determine whether you are a hidden caregiver. If you agree with more than two or three statements, there is a strong possibility that you are.

Are You a Hidden Caregiver?

You are involved in a hidden caregiving relationship if there is someone in your life who:

- Makes inappropriate requests for assistance. He may keep himself ignorant to maintain his helpless stance. ("Honey, can you tie my tie?" or "Honey, what size shirt am I?")

- Demands that her needs take priority, and invokes guilt if you try to take care of your own. Such a person sends out an implicit demand to be taken care of; if her needs are not met, she gets angry, sulks, or passively waits until you rescue her.

- Manipulates situations so he has to be taken care of. He may create emergencies or disasters, such as repeatedly locking his keys in the car, or being chronically unable to complete a shopping expedition without making at least one call home for help. (One overburdened hidden caregiver, only half in jest, reported that she wanted a license plate for her car that said RESCUE-1.)

- Is unable to provide real companionship. Because of her own neediness, she cannot tolerate the give-and-take of an adult relationship, and loses interest when she is not the center of attention.

- Evokes rage or depression in his caregiver, because the apparent reasonableness of his demands is so difficult to confront. (If you find yourself described as "irrational" or "weird" for behaving in ways that reflect your anger or depression, you may be the victim of such a person.)

The Child Whose Special Needs Emerge Over Time

Hidden caregiving may also occur when an ostensibly normal child has an as yet undiagnosed problem. Jessica was forty-three when Michael was born. From early childhood, Michael was easily frustrated and unable to control himself. Jessica wore herself out trying to keep up with him, and she finally decided, in desperation and with the support of her child's pediatrician, that a neurological evaluation was in order. To her dismay (but also relief), Jessica learned that Michael had a brain disorder that made it extremely difficult for him to organize his thoughts and turn them into coherent and logical speech. His frustration at being unable to communicate was the basis for his irritability and lack of control. Once diagnosed, he received special help and his behavior improved markedly. Jessica's relief was palpable. As the parent of an ostensibly normal child, she had run herself ragged and neglected her own needs. She felt like an incompetent parent; indeed, she appeared to be one. However, once she had been identified as the caregiver of a special needs child, she was provided with the support, information, and skills she needed to be more effective.

Reverse Role Caregiving

When a child becomes caregiver to a parent, the usual order of things—that adults take care of children—is inverted. The effect on the child can vary from discomfort and embarrassment to deep-seated resentment, distress, and a precocious sense of responsibility.

For example, one man recalled that during his early teens he spent many Friday evenings walking to local bars to find his alcoholic father, convince him to leave, and help him walk home. He still recalls the smell of alcohol and the embarrassment he felt.

An anxious and depressed ten-year-old girl described how her father could not care for himself or his family. He squandered money and injured himself in small ways. More seriously, he was unable to defend his children when an emotionally disturbed relative mistreated them. A former heroin addict who had been near death several times, the man required a lengthy hospitalization when the girl was only five. Ever since then, she felt responsible for taking care of him, and he accepted his daughter's caregiving without thinking much about it. Reluctant to let her father out of her sight for very long, she became unwilling to go to school, and was unable to visit friends without calling home.

We are not suggesting that it is wrong or bad for children to be empathic toward their parents. Such behavior lays the foundation for good social relationships in childhood and later life. But it is emotionally unhealthy for a child to feel responsible for her parent's safety or happiness. It is equally unhealthy for her to give up her own activities and ignore her own needs in deference to her parent's.

Brenda was a bright and caring twelve-year-old who spent many Saturday afternoons shopping with her mother. Although this was not how she wanted to spend her time, she knew that her mother's best friend had moved far away, and was afraid that her mother would be lonely. She avoided her friends and made plans with her mother instead. When asked how she felt about spending time this way, she shrugged and said, "It's OK, I really don't mind." However, her sad voice and droopy posture said otherwise.

Some children become their parent's confidants, burdened with information completely inappropriate for their age. James, the child caregiver of a needy mother, was told by her how little she cared for his father and how very lonely she was in her marriage. James became a surrogate spouse. Only as an adult did he realize how inappropriate it was for his mother to have used him this way.

When children are asked to take on such tasks, they are deprived of the safe and nurturing haven that is their birthright. In our view, such parental behaviors constitute a form of child abuse. Children need parents, and will do almost anything to please and protect them. By words and deeds, emotionally healthy adults reassure the child that they can take care of themselves. Disturbed and needy adults do the opposite.

Two factors make it difficult to undo this situation. First, children do not view their predicament as inappropriate because they lack a sufficiently broad frame of reference. Second, they are fiercely loyal and seldom speak out against their parents. If nothing happens over the years to call a halt to this unhealthy inversion, the child, never having been taken care of, may come to feel unworthy of care. Moreover, since people tend to recreate familiar childhood scenarios in their adult relationships, the reverse role child caregiver is at risk for becoming the hidden adult caregiver of a needy partner.

Fortunately, not all youngsters are sucked in to such dysfunctional roles. For their psychological survival, some rebel. In one instance, an emotionally drained seventeen-year-old girl left home for good in her junior year of high school in order to escape her unstable and needy mother.

The inventory that follows is designed to help you determine whether you were a reverse role caregiver as a child.

Were You a Reverse Role Caregiver?

Directions: Please respond to each of the following statements by circling Y for yes and N for no.

1. If my parent was sad or upset, I felt I had to cheer him/her up.
   Y N

2. I was often made to feel guilty if I chose to be with friends instead of with my parent. Y N

3. My parent sometimes asked me to sleep in his/her bed for company. Y N

4. When my parent hugged me, I often felt as if I wanted to break free and run. Y N

5. I sometimes felt I was my parent's partner rather than his/her child. Y N

6. When things went wrong at home, my parent looked to me to make things better. Y N

7. I often lent money to my parent. Y N

8. I was usually expected to take care of my siblings because my parents were unable to do so. Y N

9. I often wished my parents had a better relationship so I would be off the hook. Y N

10. I was often asked to side with one parent against the other.
    Y N

If you responded affirmatively to more than one or two statements, the chances are good that you were a reverse role caregiver as a child, and, consequently, you may be at risk for becoming involved in a hidden caregiving relationship as an adult.

How to Extricate Yourself

The best way to avoid the problems associated with being a hidden caregiver is to be vigilant about being drawn into this role. However, if you are already there, what can you do?

1. **Recognize that there is a problem**

If your experience coincides with what you have read in this chapter, acknowledge the fact that you are a hidden caregiver. It may be helpful to understand how you got drawn in to the role, why you were willing to continue, and whether this role gratifies your needs.

2. **Discuss the problem with your care recipient**

Explain what you believe has been going on and say how you've been feeling about it, using "I" statements (see page 57). Share your concerns, making it clear that you care for the person, but do not want to be a caregiver.

3. **Redefine your relationship**

We recommend that you and your care recipient spell out what has been expected of each of you and what you want to change. For example, if your care recipient has been relying on you because he lacks skills, encourage him to learn those skills. A husband who is completely at a loss in the kitchen can take a cooking course. A woman who cannot balance a checkbook or handle finances can read a basic book about money management or take an adult education course on personal finances at a local high school. By refusing to accept that your care recipient cannot learn, you place the responsibility back where it belongs.

If your care recipient's needs are primarily emotional, both of you may benefit from seeing a mental health professional. It's important to understand the nature of your relationship, and negotiate a more productive one. If it becomes clear that your care recipient has many issues, individual treatment might be appropriate.

CHAPTER EIGHT

WHEN YOUR CARE RECIPIENT HAS A MENTAL DISORDER

In this chapter you'll learn how to cope with the unique problems you face as the caregiver of someone who is mentally ill. Among them are feelings of shame, fear, isolation, and uncertainty about what to do or expect.

"What do I do now?" a young woman asked recently. Her husband had just been discharged from the hospital after an extravagant spending spree followed by a deep depression. "He's been diagnosed as bipolar—whatever that means," she said. "The doctor wants him to take lithium, and he doesn't want to. If he doesn't take his medication, will he get worse?"

The young woman's distress is understandable. Like so many family members charged with caring for a mentally ill person, she was ill-informed. Yet her husband had been discharged to her care. To the layperson, the term "bipolar" is meaningless. Without someone's taking the time to explain what it means and to provide at least some basic information about the treatment, the diagnosis itself leaves the caregiver knowing little more than she knew before.

In some ways, the woman was lucky. At least she was told the diagnosis. Many caregivers aren't. As a result, neither they nor their care recipients have any clear sense of what needs to be done and why, or of what precautions should be taken to prevent a relapse.

As this woman's experience indicates, anyone who provides care for a person with a mental disorder faces problems that are often quite complex. Since a comprehensive discussion of the various mental illnesses and their caregiving implications would constitute a book in itself, we will focus here on the problems most commonly encountered.

Problems Caregivers Face

The term "mental illness" has many meanings. This poses problems, as does the fact that the underlying causes of bizarre behavior are seldom clear. Still other difficulties result from the enormous emotional stresses placed on the relatives who act as caregivers for those with psychiatric diagnoses.

The Vague Meaning of "Mental Illness"

Just as a diagnosis of cancer can mean either a small, fully curable lesion, or an inoperable brain tumor, a diagnosis of mental illness can mean different things. For example:

- A mentally ill person may be quite functional or may need total care.

- Sometimes lifestyle changes, or a short course of treatment (psychotherapy and/or medication), is enough to help a person "snap out of it." For others, treatment is necessary for most of their lives.

- Even well-known terms such as "depression" and "anxiety" refer to conditions that vary widely in their nature, severity, and prognosis. For example, some anxiety disorders are chronic, others are not.

- Mental illnesses change over time. A depressed person may be suicidal at some times but not at others, and also may go into remission for no apparent reason.

- Within the psychiatric profession, there is little agreement about the origins of many mental illnesses and how best to treat them. Given the fact that the experts disagree, how are caregivers supposed to know how to help?

It's not surprising that caregivers are often confused and let down by mental health experts. Sometimes labels such as "paranoid schizophrenia" are offered as explanations of bizarre behavior. Such terms, however, provide little information and explain nothing.

The Unclear Origins of Disturbed Behavior

One difficulty in providing care for an emotionally disturbed person is that you cannot look into your care recipient's mind and understand where his symptoms are coming from. When a panic attack strikes suddenly, the lack of a clear cause can leave the caregiver feeling confused and helpless. Awareness that there is a cause, even if it's not readily apparent, and knowing how to respond to ease the sufferer's distress, make caregiving less frightening and more effective.

Caregiver Reactions to Mental Illness

Shame, fear, isolation, lack of clarity about what is expected of them, and uncertainty about the duration of the illness contribute to caregivers' dismay. Let us look at each of these in turn.

Shame

No one feels the need to hide a broken leg or to lie about a visit to the dentist. However, when it comes to mental disorders, many people do lie. They may even refuse to seek help, because of the misguided belief that they will be thought "crazy." Although modern research indicates that many mental disorders are linked to biological factors such as chemical imbalances in the brain, it is still commonly believed that these disorders are the result of a moral or personal failure.

For these same reasons, those who care for the mentally ill are often ashamed or embarrassed. Who wants to be identified as the caregiver of a crazy person? It might even be contagious! (This is no joke; some people fear that by being around people who are "weird," they will become "weird" themselves.) In many families, mental disorders are simply not discussed, or are spoken of only in hushed tones. One man reported that when his unmarried thirty-eight-year-old sister lost her job as a checkout clerk at a supermarket (a job she'd had since high school), she lost weight and began talking about ending her life. Her apartment, dirty and strewn with piles of trash, was a disaster. It was clear she could not manage on her own. "I can't leave her alone," the man said. "But I can't have her live with us, either! My wife wants no part of her. She's downright embarrassed at having a mentally ill person in the family! She's afraid for the kids. 'What if she goes crazy and hurts them?' she asked me when I suggested Sherry might come live with us. What am I supposed to do now?" The young man's dilemma was real, as were his wife's fear and embarrassment.

The problem of shame may lead to denial and even worse. Julie, a fifteen-year-old adolescent, was being sexually abused by her father. Devastated, she confided in her mother, expecting, at the very least, that she would be believed. To her dismay, she was accused of lying. Although she sought professional help, she was reluctant to bring charges against her father for fear of breaking up the family. Ultimately, she ran away from home, seeing that as the only option available to her. Other adolescents in similar situations attempt suicide or turn to drugs or alcohol to numb their pain. The root of many such responses is shame that prevents both victim and abuser from getting the help they need.

Fear

The media are quick to publicize accounts of extremely dangerous mentally ill people like the Son of Sam, John Wayne Gacey, Charles Manson, and Ted Bundy. Because of their acts, mental illness still evokes widespread fear in the minds of many.

People fear what they don't know. Although some types of mental illness may involve irrational and potentially dangerous behaviors, most do not. Many people diagnosed with a mental disorder function so well that they hardly seem ill at all. In fact, according to the National Alliance for the Mentally Ill (1999), approximately 24 percent of the population is suffering from some form of mental illness. Still, the link between mental illness and violent insanity persists.

Fear, along with uncertainty, can keep friends and relatives from visiting, or even calling. One woman, whose adolescent son became seriously depressed, spoke sadly of how his formerly close friends just stopped calling. "I understand their discomfort," she said, "but they've known Jesse for years. Is it so difficult to ask how he's doing? They act as though he no longer exists." She understood their discomfort; nevertheless, she felt hurt and angry.

Isolation and Mixed Emotions

Not long ago, *New York Times* writer Jane Brody discussed the pressures experienced by the partners of those who are chronically depressed (1998). Although her article dealt with depression exclusively, much of what she said pertains to the families of people who suffer from any serious mental illness. Partners and children are often isolated, confused, angry, and resentful. They may feel terribly frustrated because of the loss of a feeling of connection with the ill person. They may shy away from bringing friends to the house. Couples are more likely to divorce, because misunderstandings and arguments are more frequent, and resolutions more difficult to achieve. Families of psychiatric patients report they often feel as though they are walking on eggs, never quite knowing what will set the person off.

Children living at home are almost always affected by a mentally ill parent, who may be impatient, hypercritical, and emotionally unavailable. Under such circumstances, many of their needs go unfulfilled. Unexpressed resentments may show up as poor school performance, inadequate social adjustment, and various forms of acting out, such as substance abuse.

Lack of Clarity Regarding Caregiving

Because mental disorders vary widely, so does the care required. Some caregivers have only to provide a supportive environment. Others must help with even the most basic tasks. Unless you are clear about what is needed by your care recipient, you can never be sure that you are doing the most beneficial thing.

Indeterminate Length of Providing Care

Some mental disorders are transient; initially the caregiver is confronted by a very upset person who soon improves. For example, stress reactions occasioned by a natural disaster are often not prolonged, provided the victim receives help promptly. Other emotional problems are chronic. A depressed person may function adequately for years, then become depressed again as a result of some life change or stress, such as a relocation or a death in the family. When

119

providing care for someone with this condition, caregivers need to maintain vigilance to ensure that treatment is resumed when needed. Said one woman whose husband had had several depressive episodes, "This time, I was ready for it. As soon as Frank told me we would need to relocate, I started simplifying our life. I cut back on our socializing, for example. I also took responsibility for more of the day-to-day chores of running the household. I encouraged Frank to get in touch with his therapist, and reminded him that under stressful conditions, he doesn't do well. He agreed. My vigilance, and his openness and cooperation, made the relocation go pretty smoothly."

Some chronic emotional disabilities, like schizophrenia and bipolar disorder, are not only enduring, but extraordinarily disruptive. "It's a life sentence," said one woman who was responsible for her schizophrenic brother, "not only for my brother, but for me." She had been charged by her dying mother with looking after her schizophrenic brother. Divorced and in her early fifties, she had spent the better part of her life fulfilling that request. She had sacrificed her marriage, her career, and her own emotional health in the process.

How to Determine Your Role

Regardless of the type of mental disorder from which your care recipient suffers, the following questions will be helpful in evaluating your situation and determining your appropriate caregiving role. Use your answers to these questions to gauge the adequacy of the care being given, and to plan your own caregiving interventions.

1. **How well is your care recipient functioning?** Can he carry out his normal routines? For example, can he go to work? Can he fulfill his other responsibilities? What kind of help do you need to provide?

2. **How can you help meet your care recipient's needs?** Sometimes a relationship with a therapist is sufficient to meet the needs of your care recipient. In such cases, your job is just to offer support and a caring environment. At other times, more is required of you. For example, you may need to advocate on behalf of your care recipient to ensure that he gets the help he needs.

Although it is logical to turn to your care recipient's therapist for guidance and advice, that's not always possible. Because of concerns about confidentiality, some mental health professionals prefer to have little or no contact with the family. (People who are not blood relatives often have even more trouble getting information.) However, as long as your care recipient is agreeable, it is perfectly appropriate to call his therapist for guidance. In all cases, your care recipient will need to sign a release authorizing his therapist to speak with you. This is what a typical release form loks like. You will find this form in the Appendix on page 202. Feel free to reproduce it. Fill it in, and have your care recipient sign and date the form.

AUTHORIZATION TO RELEASE AND EXCHANGE INFORMATION

I **(print name)** _____

residing at **(print address and phone number)** _____

_____

hereby authorize _____

(name of therapist) to release information about my treatment

with the following individual: _____

_____ **(print your name and your**

relationship with the care recipient).

I understand that by signing this form, I am agreeing to hold

_____

(name of therapist) harmless with respect to any and all uses

to which the information he/she releases with my authoriza-

tion are put.

This authorization expires on _____ .

Signed _____ Date _____

Witness _____(waived)_____ Date _____

---

3. **Are your recipient's symptoms under control?** Are they disruptive? In extreme cases, such as when a person hears voices or imagines things that aren't real, hospitalization may be necessary.

4. **Is your care recipient dangerous?** When your recipient poses a danger to himself or others, an emergency exists requiring immediate intervention, often with the help of the police, a physician, or the patient's therapist. If this is even a remote possibility, it's best to have a plan, formulated with professional help, so that you will know what to do and whom to contact in an emergency.

Additional information is available from the organizations listed in the Resources section at the back of this book. We urge you to take full advantage of all available sources of help.

CHAPTER NINE

HELPING YOUR SPECIAL NEEDS CHILD

This chapter is for the parents of children with special needs—whether cognitive, physical, emotional, or some combination. We discuss your emotional reactions to being in this situation, and offer advice on avoiding pitfalls that can complicate your efforts to obtain appropriate educational information.

JoAnn is a thirty-seven-year-old married mother of two school-age children. Because her youngsters are learning disabled, she spends considerable amounts of time—much more than a typical parent would—overseeing their school experience. She discusses their learning problems with teachers and administrators, both informally and in the course of special meetings. She advocates on her children's behalf. She also spends a great deal of time helping both of them with homework. Despite the fact that JoAnn's activities seem not very different from that of any other parent, the extent and constancy of her work earns her the label of caregiver.

What is a special needs child? As used here, the term refers to a child classified with a physical or learning disability, emotional or behavior problem, hearing, speech, vision, or language difficulty, or a combination of challenges sufficient to interfere with academic achievement and/or social adjustment in school.

Parents of children with special needs perform extraordinary services and struggle with the same problems that beset caregivers of obviously "ill" and needy recipients. They may feel isolated, concerned, guilty, and resentful. They are often overworked, stressed, and unappreciated. Moreover, their burnout potential is high, because they must come to terms with the disappointment and anger that almost always follow the realization that their youngster may never be quite like other children. Yet, most books about special needs children (see Resources section) pay little attention to the emotional impact of the discovery that one's child is different. We will review those reactions in the next section.

The approach we recommend in this chapter is applicable not only to situations involving a classifiable or diagnosable condition, but to any requiring your support and intervention. For example, if your child is especially shy or sensitive to criticism, you may need to arrange a conference with your child's teacher or with the school psychologist to alert them to your child's problem and to request accommodation. Our suggestions can help you achieve that goal.

What It Means to Be the Parent of a Special Needs Child

From the moment a pregnancy is confirmed, most parents imagine what their child will be like. They see the youngster as healthy, "normal," and thriving. When a problem is discovered, they are faced with the death of these fantasies. The parent of a child born with a visible defect—for example, Down's syndrome—is forced to confront this reality immediately. When a child's difficulties are more subtle—emerging, perhaps, only when he or she starts school—parents may have an especially difficult time. Not only must they accept the disability, they must come to terms with being the parents of a child who appeared to be normal, but who, in fact, requires special care.

Because parents typically see their children as "a chip off the old block," a reflection of themselves, they may react to this discovery with anger, shame, and denial. Even if your child's problem is not serious, becoming the parent of a child in need of any special service most likely will require some adjustment. For example, one mother felt distressed when her child was referred to the school's speech therapist for a minor articulation disorder. She said, "I was surprised I was so upset. I remember struggling to conceal my embarrassment from other parents, and I felt ashamed of my strong reaction." Another parent, the mother of a six-year-old who had been diagnosed as learning disabled, assured one of the authors that her child was "very, very bright." She declined the suggestion that she look into a school for children with learning disabilities, just to see what they had to offer, saying, "he's not like those children." Although she expressed strong dissatisfaction with the way the local public school was handling her child's needs, she planned to allow him to remain in that school throughout the primary grades, and said that she would consider a special needs school only if he were still having difficulty by the time he was ready for junior high school.

If you have recently discovered that you are the parent of a special needs child, you should expect to have strong emotional reactions. You may very well feel angry or short-changed, and resent the additional burden thrust upon you. You may also be concerned about how well the public schools can meet your child's needs.

Here are some signs that indicate such feelings may be affecting you.

- Resistance to the idea that your child needs help

- Anger and impatience with parents who brag about their children's achievements

- Annoyance with your child for giving you this extra burden

- Anxiety when anyone speaks of your child's problems

- Feeling victimized by the unfairness of the situation— "Why me?"

- Feeling guilty that you did something to cause this problem

- Hoping that another professional will give you a more optimistic evaluation

The first step in coping with these reactions is to acknowledge their existence. Be as candid with yourself as possible. Allow time to accept your disappointment and to come to terms with your feelings. There is no shame in being human.

Second, recognize these as fairly typical reactions to an unexpected and stressful situation. Use whatever resources are available at your child's school, such as the school psychologist and learning resource specialist. Speak to other parents who have dealt with situations similar to your own, either informally or in a support group. If your child's problem will have an impact on siblings, let them know what's going on. Children are sensitive to the general family climate; many "read" their parents well, and are likely to imagine a scenario far worse than the reality. A frank discussion about what is happening can go a long way toward reducing tension and allaying fears.

Third, educate yourself about your child's problem. In the Resources section at the back of the book you'll find a list of books, websites, and organizations that can provide additional information. Use them.

How to Obtain Help for Your Special Needs Child

Until the mid 1970s, most children with learning disabilities were dismissed as stupid or unable to learn. They were given little support and few, if any, special services. In 1975, Public Law 94-142 (now known as the Individuals with Disabilities Education Act [IDEA]) came into effect. This law calls for the "least restrictive placement alternative" and mandates the preparation of a written Individual Education Plan (IEP) for each child designated as "disabled." Schools are now required to make a "free and appropriate public education" available to eligible, qualified children with a disability. In 1991, the United States Department of Education issued a Policy Clarification Memorandum expressly recognizing children with ADD (Attention Deficit Disorder) as eligible for special educational services.

Although most schools strive to provide needed remediation, shortages of funding and personnel may create difficulties. Educational administrators often complain, with some justification, that state and federal governments have imposed unfunded mandates on the public schools. By the term *unfunded mandates*, they mean that schools must provide services to learning disabled children, but receive no reimbursement for doing so. Furthermore, if a school is unable to provide the necessary services, it is up to the district to pay the child's tuition in a school that can. These costs can be substantial.

Moreover, some parents, out of concern for their child's welfare, abuse the system—coming to student conferences with lawyers and advocates, and insisting on expensive and sometimes unnecessary services. It is often less costly to accede to such unreasonable requests than to fight them in court. The unfortunate result is that parents and school personnel too often become adversaries instead of allies. Parents may be perceived by school personnel as demanding and unreasonable, while school personnel may be perceived as uncooperative and unsympathetic. To complicate matters even further, parents of special needs children sometimes displace their anger and frustrations onto school personnel, and inadvertently antagonize the very people whose support they are soliciting.

This way of proceeding does not serve the child's best interests. You can help establish a more conciliatory and cooperative way of reaching decisions that will affect your child. To do that, you must know how to proceed, what you are entitled to, and what to do if you are not satisfied. Misunderstandings are costly, counterproductive, and may delay proper intervention. For example, in one case, a very bright nine-year-old boy with suspected ADD was evaluated by the school at his mother's request. However, the school psychologist's testing failed to establish conclusively that the child had ADD. The school, following standard policy, refused to pay for retesting by an independent psychologist. The child's parents, feeling that the school should bear the cost of additional testing, did nothing. A stalemate developed. In the meantime, the child continued to fail in school. His disruption of classes and the antagonism of school personnel resulted in his detentions and suspensions. Finally, the parents had their child tested at their own expense. The new testing confirmed the suspected diagnosis, and the child began an appropriate course of medication, with dramatic results. Although the final outcome was positive, the delay in providing appropriate treatment had resulted in needless distress to everyone involved.

If You Suspect Your Child Has a Special Need

There are two ways in which a problem can come to your attention. Sometimes, a sensitive teacher will alert you to the fact that your child is experiencing difficulty. Or, you may suspect, independently, that something is wrong. For example, your child may be struggling with homework, or not getting along with classmates. In such cases, what can you do?

First, rule out any physical cause or contribution. An assessment by your child's pediatrician is a good starting point. Although you can bypass this step and go directly to the school, we do not recommend doing so. Your child's pediatrician is aware of age norms and may determine that your child's difficulty is age-appropriate and not in need of intervention at this time. Some children, for example, may develop fine motor coordination later than others, but still be well within normal limits.

Your pediatrician is also familiar with your child's history, and may be able to use it to shed light on the current situation. For example, the fall that your child had at age two may take on new significance in light of his current inability to concentrate.

If your physician does find a definite physical problem, correct it. For example, if your child needs glasses, get them. If, however, the physician suspects an abnormality that cannot be confirmed without further testing, two options present themselves. You can proceed on your own with further evaluation, e.g., if there is a suspected hearing loss, you might take your child to an audiologist. Or, you can turn to the school with your doctor's recommendation and request an evaluation. (We will discuss how to do this below.)

If the pediatric visit does not yield a plausible explanation for your child's difficulties, you have the same two options. You can explore the situation further on your own, by, for example, taking your youngster to a specialist in learning disabilities, or you can ask the school for help. When Becky was unable to concentrate in the classroom, her parents took her to her pediatrician. His examination revealed no apparent cause for her difficulty. Becky's parents requested a conference with her teacher, and they agreed to try placing her in the front of the room to see if this solved the problem. They further agreed to re-evaluate the situation in a few weeks, and see if further intervention or testing were needed.

If you decide to turn to your child's school for help at any point in the process, there are two sets of concerns you need to keep in mind. The first has to do with eligibility criteria, the second with protocol and procedures. Unfortunately, each school district uses different criteria to determine which children are entitled to special services. Therefore, when requesting an evaluation, you need to know how to proceed. Since a distinction is sometimes drawn between students who are classified as in need of special services and students who are not, you need to find out the policy in effect in your own school district. Even before approaching your child's teacher, you should call the director of special education services or the head of the committee on special education for your district.

If you are uncertain as to how to contact this person, call the office of the school superintendent. Someone there will know the person with whom you need to speak. Before calling or meeting with that person, make a list of what you need to know. During your conversation, stay focused on your questions, and write down the information you are given. You might want to include the following questions among those that you ask.

1. What kind of testing is available to students in the district?

2. What criteria are used in determining eligibility for testing?

3. What procedures must be followed to obtain testing?

4. What kinds of remediation and support services are available to students?

5. Must my child be classified as "special ed" to obtain these services?

6. What services, if any, are available to nonclassified children?

How to Work with the Politics of the System

Unfortunately, it's not enough to know your child's needs and to be willing to proceed properly and cooperatively. Neither is it enough to know how to negotiate fruitfully. You must also be familiar with the politics of the school system, including how to avoid giving offense, whom to speak to, and how to cultivate allies in key places. A basic familiarity with terminology and titles is essential. This will help you to converse meaningfully with educators and to avoid offending anyone who might otherwise be helpful. It will also keep you from feeling unsettled during school conferences. What follows is a list of key terms and what they mean.

Educational Terms You Need to Know

PPT (Pupil Planning Team)

Make up: Classroom teacher or team leader, administration representative, special education personnel (for example, school psychologist, speech therapist, and reading consultant), and one or both parents or guardians. (The make up of the Pupil Planning Team may vary slightly from one school district to another.)

Purpose: To hold scheduled conferences in order to give all parties with knowledge of the child an opportunity to review data (including test results and classroom observations) and plan strategies to be implemented by teacher(s), remediation experts, other school personnel, and parents.

What to Expect: Meetings, which are generally held during the school day, usually last about an hour. If you attend, which is advisable, you will be invited to discuss your observations, concerns, and recommendations.

Other: Follow-up session should be scheduled to evaluate the results of the implementation of the plan.

IEP (Individualized Educational Plan): A written plan, spelling out the strategies to be implemented by teacher(s), school personnel, and parents. It is arrived at during the PPT meeting.

School Psychologist: Trained in child development, psychological testing, and clinical strategies, this professional does testing and sometimes provides clinical services.

Reading Consultant: Trained in strategies to improve children's reading skills, this professional measures a student's ability to read by administering tests and other evaluation strategies, and plans remediation and enrichment programs.

School Social Worker: Trained in child development and in the impact of social context on behavior, this professional assesses family functioning and makes recommendations; may refer child and family to community resources.

Director of Pupil Personnel: This administrator oversees the work of all school personnel whose job it is to serve the needs of special children.

Language Arts Coordinator: This administrator develops curricula in reading, writing, and literature and oversees the teachers who work in these subject areas.

Math/Science Coordinator: This administrator develops curriculum and oversees the teachers who work in these subject areas.

Superintendent, Assistant Superintendent: This administrator, who is ultimately responsible for what occurs in every school in the district, is concerned with all aspects of education, including budget, personnel, and the physical plant.

Principal, Assistant Principal: This administrator, who is ultimately responsible for what occurs in the specific school over which she or he has authority, is concerned with budget, personnel, and the physical plant.

Aide: This nonprofessional implements certain aspects of IEPs under the direction of a professional such as a reading consultant.

Special: This professional teaches subjects such as art and music that are usually considered outside the standard curriculum.

Speech Therapist: This professional assesses speech and hearing problems and designs and implements therapy programs; may refer child and family to community resources.

Occupational Therapist: This professional designs and implements programs that are designed to improve basic physical skills, such as fine motor skills and eye-hand coordination

Physical Therapist: This professional designs and implements programs that are intended to overcome or minimize the impact of handicaps, such as problems with walking or balance difficulties.

Remediation Program: This is a program designed to raise a student's level of functioning; it may be implemented by professionals or aides.

It is important to follow proper protocol. Most schools have a "chain of command" you should follow when you want to express a concern or to learn about what's happening in the classroom. It is generally considered proper and courteous to approach the classroom teacher first. A note, a call, or a prearranged visit is usually the first step for presenting concerns or making requests.

If some problem exists, and reasonable attempts to solve it at the classroom level have been unsuccessful, then it's appropriate to contact the school administrator who will advise you as to the next step to take. Since the classroom is where your child "lives" while at school, it's generally best to resolve problems at this level, and to maintain a good working relationship with your child's teacher. At the end of this section (p. 136) we review the typical sequence that takes place if further intervention is necessary.

Because teachers seldom hear from parents unless there's a problem, the request for a conference is likely to arouse anxiety. Although some teachers welcome parental input and involvement of any kind, others are more guarded and possibly defensive. Still others may be dealing with difficulties of their own, which makes them more likely to be defensive and unreceptive. If you are faced with a teacher who is likely to have difficulty accepting what you have to say, you will find the following section extremely helpful.

What to Do When a Teacher Is Emotionally Fragile, Defensive, or Uncooperative

Ideally, when you arrange a conference with a teacher, you would like her/him to appreciate your concern and to work cooperatively with you. However, despite your best efforts to be tactful, a classroom teacher may feel attacked, become defensive, and be unable or unwilling to cooperate. For example, a teacher who is burnt out may be unwilling to put in any extra effort. One who has personal problems may feel too overloaded to be receptive. And an inexperienced teacher may fear that acknowledging responsibility for any problem with your child may result in the loss of her/his job.

What can you do in these situations? We advise a two-part strategy. First, when talking with the teacher, remain focused on the facts and let them speak for themselves. Do not label, judge, condemn, or attack; instead, report on what you're seeing and on what your child is saying. Second, acknowledge the positive. Emphasize all that is going well, in addition to what could be better. Following these two steps cannot guarantee success, but they are usually effective in reducing defensiveness. The following example illustrates how to use this approach.

Bonnie R was a bright but sensitive middle-school child. Unfortunately, her English teacher, Mrs. Mason, was easily irritated by her students, and often made remarks that embarrassed and intimidated them. Bonnie complained to her mother, who arranged a meeting with Mrs. Mason. When two scheduled meetings were canceled by the English teacher, Bonnie's mother called the child's guidance counselor. When the next meeting was arranged, the guidance counselor was included. Since two cancellations suggested that Mrs. Mason was either resistant or emotionally fragile, Mrs. R thought that the presence of a third, neutral party would be a good idea.

On the day of the meeting, Mrs. R brought a chart on which she had written down her daughter's complaints. The chart contained records of events and incidents, and detailed accounts of Bonnie's behaviors and Mrs. Mason's. Mrs. R. brought copies of the chart for both the teacher and the guidance counselor. The incidents were discussed in a manner that was both conciliatory and focused on clarifying what was happening in the English teacher's classroom. Mrs. R made it clear that she allowed for the possibility that Bonnie may have been responsible for some of the current difficulties.

The problem that existed between the teacher and student was discussed in detail, so that all parties were clear on what had occurred. Specific solutions were proposed, discussed, and agreed upon. Mrs. Mason said she would call Mrs. R in a month to discuss how things were going. Although Mrs. R believed that this meeting would be sufficient to handle the problem, she took the extra precaution of writing a follow-up letter to the principal (with copies to Mrs. Mason and the guidance counselor), reviewing what had been discussed and agreed upon at the meeting, and describing the proposed solutions and follow-up arrangements. Her purpose was to ensure that the principal was aware of the situation in the event that things did not work out as well as anticipated, and to provide a record that might be useful should other children have similar difficulties with this teacher.

Here is a copy of the chart that she used for the meeting; we've also included a blank chart that you might want to duplicate for your own use.

Date of Incident	What Bonnie Did	What Mrs. Mason Did
October 25	Finished assignment early and asked what to do next	Told Bonnie in an irritated voice that she should be able to figure out what to do. She later apologized for yelling at Bonnie.
November 15	Bonnie asked a question to clarify an assignment.	Mrs. Mason told Bonnie that only an idiot would not have understood the assignment.
January 17	Bonnie asked to make up some work she had missed because of a doctor's appointment.	Mrs. Mason told Bonnie that she should schedule her appointments after school, and refused to give her the work.

Date of Incident	What the Student Did	What the Teacher Did

General Principles for Meeting with School Personnel

Here is a summary of the general principles to use when meeting with your child's teacher and other school personnel.

1. **Let the facts speak for themselves.** Whenever possible, focus on behaviors that you have observed personally, or have been able to verify. Failing that, try to be as objective as possible, since a child's reports may be distorted or exaggerated. Avoid attacking or blaming, and try to create a cooperative relationship. Focus on the common problem. For example, "I know Bonnie has been misbehaving in class, and I'm sure that upsets you. But from what I can gather, she seems to have the impression that you don't like her. Do you have a sense of why she might feel this way?" Talk about what is actually happening and what you would like to have happen. For example, "I really want my son to enjoy science. He seems afraid to ask questions in front of his peers, or to admit that he doesn't understand. I really wish it were possible for him to feel safe enough to ask questions or to admit he's confused. What do you think we can do about this?"

   In preparation for this aspect of your meeting, it would be a good idea to use the table we provided on page 134. or a similar written document. Since "in the heat of battle" you are likely to become anxious, lose your focus, and forget much of what you planned to say, using such a table, with copies for all the people at the meeting, should both strengthen your arguments and reduce your anxiety.

2. **Emphasize the positive.** You may not be feeling very appreciative of the teacher in view of your child's problem with him or her. However, no matter how angry you may feel, there is little to be gained by threats or an antagonistic attitude. Your awareness of the demands of teaching and your expression of appreciation for hard work and caring will go a long way toward securing the teacher's perception of you as an ally, not an adversary.

When the School Must Provide Special Services

If more is needed than a conference with your child's classroom teacher, the formal referral process begins. Here are the usual steps in that process:

- Once a problem has been identified, school personnel prepare a document requesting formal evaluation or screening. (The parents must give their consent for the evaluation to proceed.) At this point, professionals such as the school psychologist and reading specialist may become involved. Then, formal testing is initiated.

- The professionals' findings are reviewed, along with teacher reports and anecdotal records. As a group, these professionals decide whether your child qualifies for special services. An Individualized Educational Program (IEP) is created, and parental consent for participation is obtained.

- In some school districts, these recommendations are passed on to the district committee on special education for final approval. After all necessary approvals have been obtained, the child begins to participate in the program. The IEP is reviewed annually, with parental participation, and a new program is developed for the following year.

- The child's parents are involved, by law, at every step of the process. Your input is a valuable component in the decisions that are made. You are, in fact, part of a caregiving team.

A Final Note

As with other types of caregiving, much of what you accomplish depends on your own emotional well-being. Because meeting the needs of a special needs child is such a natural extension of normal parenting, you may not realize that the effort you are expending is unusual, even extraordinary. You need to observe the same cautions as all caregivers. For example, self-care is essential, as are acknowledging your feelings and taking active steps to prevent burnout. Children are generally sensitive to their parents' feelings, and they are quick to feel responsible or at fault. Therefore, it is especially important to give yourself appropriate outlets for the stress and frustration you will probably experience. By taking care of yourself, you will be in a much stronger position to take effective and compassionate care of your child.

CHAPTER TEN

LONG-DISTANCE
CAREGIVING

In this chapter we offer practical solutions and guidance on handling the problems posed by long-distance caregiving.

When family members lived near each other, the difficulty of providing care for aging and ill relatives was not complicated by physical distance. However, in today's mobile society, as educational and career opportunities beckon, adult children may scatter far and wide, and at retirement parents may move to gentler climates.

For these reasons, more and more caregivers are providing care from afar. This is especially true when the care recipients are elderly—parents, grandparents, or other older relations. According to a 1997 survey by the National Council on Aging and the Pew Charitable Trust (*The Washington Post*, March 23, 1997), nearly 7 million people help care for an older relative or friend who lives more than an hour's travel time away.

Many of these caregivers also work for a living. According to the Family and Work Institute (Work and Family Life, September, 1998), 25 percent of American workers have eldercare responsibilities, and 42 percent expect to assume such responsibilities within the next few years. These caregiving responsibilities necessitate taking off, on average, one work day per month, as well as occasionally having to leave work early or arrive late.

What Is a Long-Distance Caregiver?

There is no simple and workable definition of the term "long-distance caregiver." In the Pew Charitable Trust survey cited earlier, long-distance caregivers are defined as primary caregivers who live more than an hour away from their care recipients. This definition, however, is not particularly useful, because it groups together the caregiver living in New York whose mother lives in Connecticut with the caregiver living in New York whose mother lives in California. Although both have something in common (neither is "on site"), the greater the distance, the greater the potential for inconvenience and distress. For example, a woman living in Europe, whose elderly and failing mother lives in New York, has to deal with the reality of being unable to book a flight during key vacation periods, no matter what crisis has occurred.

We will first deal with problems that are common to all long-distance caregivers, and then with those that apply primarily to caregivers living at distances that involve at least an overnight stay.

Problems Faced by All Long-Distance Caregivers

By necessity, visits to your care recipient simply take more time than they would if he or she lived close by. You cannot drop in on Mom on your way home from work, nor can you easily accompany her to her doctor's appointment. Rather, each visit represents a major disruption in your own and your family's life. If you have young children, you must arrange for child care. If you are employed, you must take time off. And the time and effort that it takes to make these accommodations may be more draining and time-consuming than the actual visit. Long-distance caregivers typically must contend with the following:

Fatigue. Travel is tiring. "I drive an hour and a half to visit my mother," said one fifty-six-year-old woman. "By the time I arrive, I'm beat. Then I have to start shopping, cooking, and doing laundry. By the time the day ends, you could scrape me off the floor. Then I drive an hour and a half to get home, where my husband and children expect me to pick up where I left off!"

Emotional stress. When you're not "on site," you can't see what is happening. You can't verify the reports of others. "If only I could see with my own eyes what's going on," said a teacher whose mother had had a stroke. "I'd know whether my mother's reports of abusive behavior were true." In addition, being far away results in a distinct feeling of loss of control. "If I were with my father," said one woman who'd received upsetting news about the man's refusal to take medication, "I'd be able to talk with him and find out what the problem is. Telephone calls just aren't adequate!"

Work stress. Although many employers are understanding and flexible where caregiving is concerned, there are limits. "I'm constantly weighing my own needs for time against my boss's demands," said one woman. "I don't want to take advantage, but I wonder just how much leeway I have." The reality is that repeated absences, lateness, and early departures do affect one's standing with peers and superiors, as do lengthy personal calls from the office and other such distractions.

Special Problems You Face When You Are Very Far Away

Long-distance caregivers who live a great distance from their care recipients have additional difficulties.

All of the problems described above are magnified. If you are gone for several days, your child-care arrangements and employment accommodations are necessarily more complex than if you were gone for several hours. Your homecoming, too, is likely to be more problematic. Even relatively trivial matters, such as accumulations of laundry and mail, are potential stressors. Your fatigue is greater when you have spent seven hours on a plane than when you have spent two hours in a car. And, a distressed child or spouse who feels abandoned may have to be comforted or placated.

Expenses. Typically, long-distance caregivers accumulate huge phone bills. Transportation, particularly if airfare is involved, is also expensive. Although it may seem uncaring to consider cost when someone's health or well-being is at stake, many families cannot readily absorb the additional financial burden. "How can I weigh my mother's needs against dollars?" one man asked us recently. "Sure, I can fly back to her, but does the situation warrant the expense? In an emergency, I'd fly out to her at a moment's notice. But what, exactly, is an emergency? I want to take care of her, but I also have to be practical!"

Travel preparations. Before you leave, you must pack and make appropriate plane, car, or hotel reservations. You must be sure you have all needed information with you, and sufficient funds. And you must do all this while coping with the stress of whatever has occurred to make your visit necessary at this time. There is a checklist on pages 148–149 to guide you when you must travel quickly to reach your care recipient.

The Choice to Provide Care from Afar

Although it would be ideal to be able to choose whether or not to become a long-distance caregiver, at times you may have no option. Assume, for example, that your seventy-two-year-old mother lives in Illinois, while you and your family live on the East Coast. If she falls one day and requires emergency medical care, you have no choice but to respond. However, there is a difference between short-term crisis intervention and managing nonemergency care on a regular basis from far away. Later in the chapter, we provide specific advice on coping with emergency long-distance caregiving. Now, however, we want to focus on the variables that determine whether non-emergency long-distance care is feasible.

Factors Determining Whether Long-Distance Caregiving Is Feasible

As a potential long-distance caregiver, you need to be concerned with your own situation as well as that of your care recipient. Both of these should guide you when deciding whether to take on the responsibilities of long-distance caregiving.

Caregiver Considerations

Before deciding to become a long-distance caregiver, ask yourself the following questions:

1. *Since long distance caregiving requires travel, can you tolerate the physical fatigue that may result?* If you must drive to your care recipient, can you do so for the amounts of time required? Can you drive comfortably at night? Under poor travel conditions? If you must use public transportation, can you sit for the required long periods of time? Can you walk the distances often demanded of travelers in airports and other facilities?

2. *How will your decision impact on your family responsibilities?* One woman began making regular weekend trips to visit her elderly parents who needed her help with routine tasks like shopping and doing laundry. Her husband and two teenage children were initially gracious and understanding. However, after several months, they became intolerant of her absences. Family arguments became more common, and—at times—when she returned home she was greeted by stony silence. Enraged at her family's rudeness, she became sullen and noncommunicative herself. The situation deteriorated until a relative suggested this family needed to get help. "I realized when we began seeing a therapist that I'd just assumed my husband and children would understand," said the woman. "They loved my parents, too, so I didn't think my absences would become an issue." She was angry with her spouse and children, and had not realized the burden her decision had placed on them. If the time and energy you spend in long-distance caregiving jeopardizes the well-being of your family, that option may simply not be viable.

3. *What about work responsibilities?* If you work, even parttime, you must factor that commitment into your decision. Can you meet your care recipient's needs without jeopardizing your job? "Taking care of my sister is tough enough when I have to field calls from home," said one woman who had been the caregiver for her mentally ill sibling for many years. "But when she or her therapist calls me at work to tell me about one crisis or another, I just can't get my work done."

   Another woman lost her job after taking too many days off to visit her ailing father who lived three hours away. "I don't blame my boss," she said with resignation. "I was taking a day off almost every week!" In cases like these, where long-distance caregiving imposes burdens that are inconsistent with working for a living, you must consider your priorities and responsibilities before making a decision.

4. *Can you afford the financial cost of being a long-distance caregiver?* As noted previously, long-distance caregivers typically absorb considerable out-of-pocket expenses when they assume their task. Although initially this may not be an issue, over time it may create serious resentments.

5. *Can you afford the emotional cost?* While some degree of emotional stress, uncertainty, and guilt typically accompanies caregiving, these feelings are exacerbated when you provide

care from afar. Feelings of helplessness are heightened as you rely on others to provide actual hands-on care. Regardless of the adequacy of the care, long-distance caregivers often feel guilt and concern when they are not there to deliver the care personally. A typical reaction was expressed by one woman, whose mother was in a nursing facility in a distant state. "My mother's social worker says she loves mother and enjoys taking her out to lunch and on other outings. I suppose I should be grateful for that," she said, "but I feel so guilty. I should be the one taking mother out!"

6. *How effectively can you communicate with others?* Despite the availability of the telephone, paging devices, answering machines, email, faxes, voice mail and other up-to-the-minute communication modalities, conversation over distances is rarely efficient or easy. Delays and misunderstandings are common. Sometimes, because of the distance, your concerns are discounted by professionals and others who may assume that if you really cared, you'd be there. Calls can be ignored. "I called my father's doctor four times yesterday," said one man. "By the fourth time, his receptionist was annoyed and rude to me. And the doctor never called me back! I was frantic! I felt I was between a rock and a hard place. I need the doctor's good will, and his staff's cooperation, too. If I antagonize them, I lose. But if I can't get through to him, I lose, too!" Unfortunately, this man's experience is typical. Unless you are assertive enough to deal with such dilemmas, and have the resilience to cope with them, long-distance caregiving may not be for you.

Care Recipient Considerations

Although it is important to consider your own temperament and circumstances in making the decision to become a long-distance caregiver, it is equally important to weigh the needs, temperament, and preferences of your care recipient. We will review each of these below.

1. *What are your care recipient's needs?* Are his/her current living conditions safe and convenient? What, if anything, needs to be arranged for or changed? For example, one eighty-two-year-old man who lived in the Northeast did fine during three seasons of the year, but each winter he had to shovel snow to get to his car. One day, he fell while shoveling, and severely injured himself. It was only then that his daughter,

who lived in Florida, realized that his safety could no longer be assumed during the winter months.

Another aspect of your care recipient's needs has to do with the level of care he or she requires. Disability experts have devised ways of simplifying this process. They have grouped day-to-day activities into two sets of categories. The first set is called "Activities of Daily Living." These activities include the following: bathing, dressing, using the toilet, walking safely, eating, and maintaining continence. To live independently people must be able to perform these activities. Those who cannot require intensive help, best provided by professionals in a nursing home setting.

The second set is called "Incidental Activities of Daily Living." These are important, but not essential: using the telephone, getting to places beyond walking distance from home, managing money (paying bills, for example), doing housework (including laundry and cooking), taking medications correctly, and performing minor "handyman" tasks such as changing a light bulb. Often, these activities can be provided by "in-home" helpers. In arranging for that, you would need to consult with professionals to determine what services are available. If your care recipient is elderly, one good way to do that is to contact the National Association of Area Agencies on Aging, (202) 296-8130, to get the address and phone of the nearest Area Agency on Aging. That organization can point you to home-health and social service agencies in the area. (If your care recipient is not elderly, a call to the state Department of Social Services will yield similarly helpful information.)

Another consideration is the stability or instability of your care recipient's condition. If it is tenuous or subject to rapid or unpredictable deterioration, providing care from afar may be unwise. For example, a diabetic who cannot monitor his blood levels effectively can quickly reach a crisis state. A person with poor balance is in constant risk of falling. In cases such as these, on-site caregiving is crucial. Unless you can pay for round-the-clock care, and be certain such care is provided responsibly and competently, you cannot do conscientious caregiving from afar.

2. *What is your care recipient's temperament?* Your care recipient's personality cannot be ignored. Some care recipients are comfortable depending on others; some are not. Some value independence over security; others have the opposite priori-

ties. One ninety-year-old woman refused to leave her small ranch home despite ill health. Her son insisted that she was no longer safe living on her own. "What would happen if you fall?" he asked. "Who would help you? Who would even know?" The woman solved the problem by contacting her physician and arranging for an emergency response system—a pendant she wore around her neck— to enable her to summon help if she needed it. "My son worries too much," she said. "I got this button so he could relax."

Unfortunately, some care recipients are not at all comfortable accepting help from nonfamily members, especially from members of racial and ethnic groups with which they are not familiar. Factors such as upbringing and past experiences play a major part in the willingness to accept this kind of help. Also, the "right" or "wrong" mix of personalities may ultimately determine whether your care recipient and his helper get along or not.

3. *What are your care recipient's preferences?* Self-determination (the right to make all choices about how one lives) must also be honored whenever possible. Your care recipient may not want to relocate, or to accept the help you offer. In one case, a woman who lived in Boston was responsible for the care of her mother who lived in Virginia. In Virginia, the eighty-year-old mother had a network of friends and neighbors acquired over many years. They looked after her and provided social contact. Hard of hearing and nearly blind, she felt accepted by them.

When she became ill, her daughter decided, against the mother's wishes, to move her to Boston. Within a matter of weeks, the mother's home was placed on the market, its contents sold, and the elderly woman moved into an apartment near her daughter. Angry at the loss of her home and cherished possessions, isolated from her friends, the eighty-year-old complained and argued with her daughter constantly.

The daughter, well-meaning though she was, had violated the principle of self-determination. So long as a care recipient is competent, regardless of age or physical condition, she/he has the ultimate say in how and where she/he will live. Although this principle is generally accepted in the helping professions and in law, it is not without controversy. Problems arise when, for example, a care recipient insists on living alone when he is clearly incapable of doing do, even with at-home help. In cases like these, a care recipient may have to be declared incompetent for his own protection. If you face this situation in your own family, consult an attorney experienced in such matters and proceed according to that professional's recommendations.

When Long-Distance Caregiving Is Viable: Two Key Tasks

Assuming that both your situation and your care recipient's make nonemergency long-distance caregiving a viable option, you must first arrange for and oversee day-to-day care. This involves determining your care recipient's initial needs, staying informed about gradual and anticipated changes in your care recipient's condition, and making adjustments as necessary.

Secondly, you must prepare to cope with sudden changes and medical emergencies. This requires advance preparation and planning, including developing a network of emergency contacts and surrogate caregivers.

Help with Arranging for and Managing Day-to-Day Care

As was said previously, the first step in arranging for day-to-day care is to find out exactly what your care recipient needs. This process, called assessment, is ongoing. As a person's condition changes (for example, as a person ages, or as a disease progresses), it's necessary to re-assess and to plan for support services that are responsive.

To demonstrate how the process of assessment works, we'd like to walk you through a hypothetical case. Imagine that one day while you're at work you receive a phone call and learn that your seventy-three-year-old widowed mother, who lives five hours away, has been involved in a minor auto accident. She is not seriously injured, and requires only an overnight stay in the hospital. Nevertheless, she needs some help until her injuries heal. The hospital discharge planner can arrange for a home health aide to cook, do laundry, and attend to day-to-day tasks for a week. That certainly solves the immediate problem. However, the discharge planner expresses some concerns about your mother's ability to continue to live independently. She is frail and seems a little confused about how to manage some of the responsibilities of a homemaker.

The accident is, in reality, a wake-up call: your mother is not getting any younger, and is living alone. You realize you must begin thinking about the future. You find yourself pondering questions such as: What needs does Mom have? Is her home as safe as it can be for her? What would help her continue to manage to live on her own? Can she cook, shop? What can she not do? When you start thinking in this manner, considering your mother's current and future needs, you have begun the process of assessment.

Previously we discussed the two categories of activities that disability experts have devised for assessing a person's ability to function independently. They are the "Activities of Daily Living" (such as bathing and walking) and the "Incidental Activities of Daily Living" (such as doing laundry and changing a light bulb). Once you have determined that your mother can perform all necessary "ADLs," the next task is to locate helpers who can provide assistance with the "IADLs."

There are several national for-profit companies that specialize in providing home-health assistance. Most companies employ people capable of providing care that ranges from unskilled, such as housework, to skilled, such as dressing wounds. Look in the Yellow Pages or call a hospital in your care recipient's area for the names and phone numbers of local home-health agencies.

There are local and regional organizations, such as the Visiting Nurse Associations that offer similar kinds of help. Information about VNAs all over the country is available through the Visiting Nurse Association of America, (617) 426-5555. Alternatively, call the county medical society, a local social service agency, or your care recipient's state Department of Social Services to learn about these.

Finally, if your mother were to have a particular injury or illness (if, for example, she were paraplegic as a result of an accident, or if she had Alzheimer's), you could contact an organization with a specialized interest, such as the National Spinal Cord Injury Hotline (800-526-3456) or the Alzheimer's Foundation (800-272-3900). Lists of organizations such as these are available from your local library. There are also organizations that have been created to serve as resources for family caregivers. Two of these—both very useful clearing houses of information and sources of support—are the National Caregiving Foundation, (703) 356-8417, and the National Family Caregivers Association, (301) 942-6430.

If you are unable to perform your own assessment, locate resources, or arrange for care, you'll need to hire a professional to do these tasks for you. There are several useful sources of information. One is the National Association of Professional Geriatric Care Managers, 1604 North Country Club Road, Tucson, AZ, 85716; (520)-881-8008. Despite the name of this organization, "geriatric" care managers serve a range of disabled people. Each care manager must meet very specific qualification criteria, so you can assume a basic level of familiarity with the problems of the disabled and some expertise in locating and monitoring services.

Preparing for Emergencies

Emergencies happen, no matter how carefully you arrange for care and no matter how conscientiously you monitor it. Whether you visit or not, whether you call regularly, whether you are a superior or an inferior caregiver, there will almost always be a time when the unexpected occurs: a fall, a stroke, a mishap in the basement workshop. How can you most effectively deal with these emergencies?

There is no single "right" course of action or way of coping. Emergencies differ. Personalities differ. Nevertheless, there is one rule that applies to all cases: Do your thinking ahead of time, when you can think clearly. Plan for emergencies, and prepare for them.

These are the essential elements of an emergency plan:

Arrange in advance for an emergency contact near your care recipient—a neighbor or a relative—and know how to reach that person. Make sure the person is willing to check on your care recipient in a possible emergency, regardless of the time and on short notice. Keep the name of the contact person with you at all times.

- If your recipient's condition is very precarious, keep a bag packed and ready to go. This gives you one less thing to think about.

- If you have children, make arrangements for child care so that, if necessary, you can leave at a moment's notice.

- If air travel, other public transportation, or car rental will be required, keep phone numbers handy.

- Keep some cash on hand. You may need a credit card for certain purposes (to charge an airline ticket or to rent a car), so be certain you have one.

- Prepare a list of contact numbers to take with you so that when you arrive at your care recipient's residence, you will have the names and phone numbers of key people such as her physician and other health-care team members, her aide, and a neighbor. This will save you the time and stress of gathering this information under duress.

- Bring everything you're likely to need. For example, if it will be necessary to make calls to relatives, bring the appropriate numbers. If you will need to pay your recipient's bills, bring a checkbook. If your emergency visit requires that you cancel pending plans, bring the information needed.

- Your job, once you arrive, is to assess the situation, attend to your care recipient's needs as an "on-site" caregiver would, and make arrangements that will allow you to stay on top of the situation once you return home.

- To make sure that you don't forget anything when you have to leave on short notice, fill out the chart below and keep it handy.

Preparing for an Emergency	
Category	**Specifics**
Emergency contacts	Neighbor's phone number: _____ Physician's phone number: _____ Other phone numbers: _____ _____
Child care arrangements	Babysitter's phone number: _____ Other: _____ Meals: _____

Transportation	Airline phone number: _____
	Bus or train phone number: _____
	Car rental phone number: _____
	Other: _____

Other Preparations to Make

	Yes	No

1. My emergency luggage:
    Clothing:
 	
    Toiletries:
 	
    Medication:
 	
    Personal Scheduler:
 	
    Other:		

2. Have I arranged for work coverage?		
3. Other:		

Making a commitment to provide care from afar is a serious decision. To do so without weighing your care recipient's needs—for safety, comfort, and convenience—is a mistake. Similarly, making the decision without considering your own needs—for example, your family and work responsibilities, as well as your own emotional and financial limits—is foolhardy. If your decision is to go forward, then make full use of all the resources available to you.

CHAPTER ELEVEN

WHEN YOUR CARE RECIPIENT DIES

In this chapter we provide practical guidance on preparing for and coping with the death of your care recipient.

When your care recipient is elderly or terminally ill, you must face the reality of impending death. Difficult as this is, it serves a valuable purpose. Knowing that your care recipient will die gives both of you time to prepare and use this time for healing past wounds and for saying good-bye.

Not long ago we received the following letter from a former client. "My mother died three weeks ago," he wrote, "so I'm no longer a caregiver. But I wanted to thank you for your guidance during the time I spent agonizing over whether to move here to be with her. It was definitely the right choice. Over the past six months, we spent more time together than we had for many years, and we used it to say things that needed to be said. And although I was sad when she died, I'm glad we had time for a proper good-bye."

Preparing for Your Care Recipient's Death

As your care recipient approaches death, you need to know his wishes for his final days and hours. Most people find the prospect of asking these kinds of questions distressing, even if there are compelling reasons to do so. Death is among the most difficult of topics to discuss; no one likes to experience a loss or to be reminded of his own mortality. However, talking about death is the best way for you and your care recipient to come to terms with it, and talking about it provides many of the following emotional benefits:

- It is a chance to say good-bye to your care recipient and gives both of you a sense of closure.

- It is an opportunity to feel the satisfaction that comes from having fulfilled a final responsibility.

- It puts the care recipient's mind at ease, knowing that his wishes are clear and his affairs are in order.

Talking about death need not be morbid. Often the dying person wants to talk, but senses the discomfort of others and remains silent. If you feel that this is happening, take the initiative and bring up the subject. It's often easiest to start off with a structured question. For example, you might say, "Dad, you're pretty sick, and I'm not sure I know what you want if your doctor asks me about life support. Can we discuss it?" His response will tell you whether he's ready to talk. Once you open the door, you should be able to bring up other issues, such as do not resuscitate orders (DNR), and eventually you will get to his feelings about dying. You can use this time to share your own feelings as well. The more you can accomplish at this point, the easier your mourning will be after his death. Plan to have many short discussions, since they are likely to be emotionally draining for both of you.

Discussion of end-of-life care will almost certainly include advance directives such as a living will, a written statement of what your care recipient wants done to preserve his life. Does he want his life preserved at all costs, taking full advantage of medical technology? Or does he want only to be kept comfortable? You need to know this to ensure that health-care providers will respect his wishes. Copies of the necessary forms, along with directions for completing them, are available from members of your care recipient's health-care team, your local hospital, or from the national organization, Choice in Dying (1-800-989-WILL).

Another question that needs to be addressed is who will make treatment decisions when your care recipient is no longer able to make his preferences known. Preferences about funeral and burial arrangements also need to be made clear, as do wishes about organ donation. It's important to know if your care recipient has prepared a will and where it's located. (If no will exists, and your care recipient is legally competent, encourage him to write one before he dies.)

It is wise to document the information you get from your discussions and to keep other family members informed. This avoids the appearance of collusion or secrecy, and reduces the likelihood of disagreements down the road.

Coping with Your Care Recipient's Death

Accepting a death means coming to terms with it, closing the door on that person's life, and going on with your own. Regardless of the circumstances, death is invariably difficult to accept. First of all, it is a permanent loss. Once someone dies, you no longer have that person in your life. Thanatologists, people who study death and its effects on survivors, have identified several variables that affect how people react to another person's death. Some of these are discussed below.

How close were you and what was the nature of the attachment? Obviously, people are less likely to be strongly affected by the death of a distant cousin than by that of a spouse. As a caregiver you were, of necessity, closely involved with your care recipient. If he suffered from a chronic illness, you probably saw him struggle, rally, and then sink again. You saw the hope, the despair, and the fear. With such prolonged and intimate contact, an emotional attachment can become very strong.

How important was this person to your feelings of security, well-being, and self-esteem? The more you relied on this person to maintain a sense of your worth and value, the greater the difficulty you are likely to experience at his or her death.

How did the person die? Was the death expected or was it sudden? Did it occur because of natural causes, accident, or suicide? This factor is so important that the next section of this chapter is devoted to a more complete discussion.

Where was the deceased in the lifecycle at death? An "untimely" death, such as that of a child or a young mother, is especially difficult to accept. On the other hand, the death of a ninety-year-old who has led a full life is seldom tragic.

How have you coped with prior losses? How do you cope with stress in general? How easy is it for you to talk about your feelings?

Do you become depressed easily? Your previous experience with loss may indicate something about how you will cope with this one.

What kind of emotional support can you expect from others? Can you find comfort in your religious or humanitarian beliefs and in the rituals surrounding death? Can your family and community see you through the crisis, or are you isolated?

What simultaneous stressors are you experiencing? Other events going on in your life can affect how well you cope. Have you just lost a job? Do you have an ill child? Are other life changes draining your energy?

When your care recipient dies, you may feel a loss of meaning and purpose, and may even experience the death as a personal failure. If you have been a caregiver for a long time, your life may have come to revolve around providing care. Sadness and anger are common responses. So are guilt, loneliness, self-reproach, anxiety, shock, yearning, and numbness. Many caregivers, however, are surprised to find that they also feel relief; then they struggle with feelings of guilt about the relief they feel.

The Way Your Care Recipient Dies

The way your care recipient dies affects your reactions. Knowing that your father has died of old age may not mitigate your sense of loss, but there is something about a person's having lived a long time that makes death more acceptable There is also some comfort in seeing a loved one die after having suffered a great deal, where death represents a surcease from pain.

When, however, there are no mitigating circumstances, when a death is unexpected or was preventable, the emotional toll on the caregiver can be enormous. We'll now examine several different circumstances, each of which can make coping with the death of a care recipient especially difficult.

Sudden and/or Unexpected Death

Sasha's death occurred completely out of the blue. The eighteen-year-old had sustained a serious but not life-threatening injury in an auto accident and was recovering well at home. When she developed an infection following routine surgery, no one was alarmed. Within a day, however, it was apparent that a serious problem had arisen. Sasha's temperature spiked rapidly. She lost consciousness soon afterward and was rushed to a nearby hospital. The nurses and doctors did all they could to lower her temperature and treat the infection. When they were unsuccessful, she was transferred to the Intensive Care Unit where, despite heroic efforts, she died a few hours later.

Sasha's loss was especially tragic because she had been doing so well. Her family, at first numb and disbelieving, needed to understand what had happened. They were given straightforward explanations by the medical personnel at the hospital. Nevertheless, they could not comprehend the fact that she had died despite the most up-to-date medical care available. Their tremendous sadness quickly turned into rage. The family blamed the doctor, the hospital, and the nursing staff for their daughter's death.

Sasha's family's response was not unusual. Because it is so difficult to accept a sudden and unexpected death, survivors typically feel numb and dazed. "Sasha's death seemed completely unreal to me," her mother recalled. "I knew what was happening, but I didn't really believe it."

Survivors want to understand what occurred and why. When no "satisfactory" explanation can be provided, their acute sadness can turn into rage very quickly. If the death occurs at home while the patient is under the care of a family member, that caregiver is likely to blame herself. Unfortunately, others in the family may do the same. If home-care workers are involved (a visiting nurse or an aide, for instance), they might be blamed. Often it takes many months for these reactions to subside. Since there was no time to prepare for the death, there may be a sense of lack of closure, accompanied by strong feelings of guilt, shame, and failure. "It's all my fault!" cried one woman whose son died unexpectedly during a basketball game. "I never dreamed he had a heart problem. I should have insisted that we see our own doctor before I let him join the team."

Caregivers often express deep regret, and a closely related tendency to second-guess themselves ("If only I had . . ."). Many wish they could turn the clock back and have another chance, as though they should have known better. In so doing, they increase their burden of sadness and guilt.

Avoidable or Preventable Death

Murray, an eighty-year-old diabetic, was injected with insulin by his family doctor during a routine office visit. By the evening of that day, Murray was not feeling well and lay down to rest. When Betty, his wife, was unable to rouse him, she called the doctor. Despite her mounting concern, she did nothing until the doctor called back a half hour later.

By the time she was told to call 911, Murray had gone into insulin shock, and he died on the way to the hospital.

When a death is preventable, the caregiver is likely to feel guilty. Although Betty's response—to call the physician—was not inappropriate, she failed to convey the urgency of her situation or to call 911 immediately. Had she done either, her husband's life might well have been saved. Betty's experience illustrates how personality traits may interfere with judgment. By nature a passive and dependent woman, Betty was not used to making decisions and even the sight of her husband's limp body was not sufficient to spur her to action.

Another woman, whose husband was bleeding internally, accepted a doctor's appointment for the following week instead of insisting on an appointment for that very day. When her husband went into cardiac arrest, she said, sadly, "I told them that he was bleeding, but assumed that since they didn't make a big deal out of it, it wasn't anything we should worry about."

Both of these caregivers proceeded with good intentions, yet their inability to assert themselves played a part in the death of their spouses.

Death Caused by the Caregiver

Even more wrenching than a preventable death are those instances in which a caregiver causes a death. Sometimes, accidents happen. Janet was driving her mother to a doctor's appointment when her brakes failed. Although her car's airbags deployed, her mother's frail bones were unable to withstand the impact and her chest was crushed. Janet suffered from profound guilt for many months after her mother died, in spite of the fact that it had been an accident that no one could have foreseen.

Sometimes mistakes are made, as when the wrong medication is administered. Other times, caregivers make errors of judgment. In one case, a depressed care recipient assured his sibling that he would be fine. "I believed him," said his sister, later. "So I went home." Tragically, when she returned, she found her brother's body. He had committed suicide.

Such experiences, profoundly traumatic in themselves, may be made more difficult by other bereaved relatives who blame the caregiver. As mentioned previously, no one can be expected to foresee all possible outcomes. Even professionals may have to make "judgment calls" at times, and they are sometimes wrong. Since errors are more likely to be made when a caregiver is distracted or fatigued, self-care becomes more than a luxury for the caregiver. It may also be a lifesaver for the care recipient.

Suicide

There are different kinds of suicide. Planned suicide, as when someone in intractable pain wishes to die by his own hand, often requires the cooperation of close family members and friends. And, even if carried out alone, its effects on others are often carefully considered, as the following case illustrates.

When Barbara committed suicide, she left a note to her family in which she explained that she saw no point in living with multiple sclerosis any longer. She was afraid to discuss her plans with her family for fear of burdening them. "I am truly sorry for your pain, but I hope you will understand," she wrote. Barbara stored up a lethal medication and deliberately overdosed during the night.

In such cases, the suicide is a deliberate act, motivated by a desire to avoid further suffering. Sometimes, however, suicide is not premeditated, but is an impulsive act, carried out in a moment of acute rage or despair. For example, one young man became totally distraught after learning that his cancer, long in remission, had reappeared. He left the doctor's office, walked angrily to his car, sped away, and seconds later crashed into a tree.

When a care recipient commits suicide, his caregiver typically feels abandoned, betrayed, and extremely angry. Said Craig, the husband of Barbara, whose story we told above, "I feel like my wife was playing me for a fool. Here I was doing my best to keep her alive, while she was planning her death. I just can't forgive her—or myself—for that!" Another person remarked that his father's suicide felt like a personal rejection. "If he loved me enough he would never have killed himself."

Often, caregivers and other family members feel acute shame because of the stigma attached to suicide. These feelings are reflected in a reluctance to talk about the death. Sometimes the family attempts to keep the suicide a secret, resulting in an additional burden as well as deprivation of support. In addition, caregivers are likely to experience feelings of failure and guilt. Barbara's husband berated himself, feeling that he should have monitored her medication more closely.

It is also not unusual for the relatives of a suicide victim to fear for themselves. "Will I kill myself, too?" asked a teenage boy after a depressed uncle committed suicide. He was especially concerned because there had been two other suicides on his father's side of his family. Although he was assured that depression, when treated, does not inevitably lead to suicide, the fact remains that proximity to a suicide is indeed a risk factor. Whenever a suicide occurs, especially that of a young person, professional intervention is highly advisable to prevent "copycat" suicides. Open discussion, without shame or blame, and emphasis on better ways of coping, may prevent one tragedy from turning into several.

No discussion of death would be complete without mentioning physician-assisted suicide. During the 1990s, physician Jack Kevorkian has sparked controversy by administering lethal doses of medications to help people end their lives. Kevorkian has been treated as an outcast by the medical community and by others in the "right-to-die" movement. He is a pathologist with a penchant for the bizarre (his ghoulish paintings have been the subject of more than one critical essay), and is neither a likable personality nor an eloquent spokesman for his cause. Although many family members of those he helped to kill themselves have expressed their gratitude, Kevorkian's "in your face" style has gained him many more enemies than friends. As of this writing, he has been found guilty of second-degree murder in a state court and sentenced to ten to twenty-five years in jail. An appeal is pending.

Getting Over a Death

Surviving the death of your care recipient involves working your way through the four stages of the mourning process.

Numbness. The intensity of this feeling may be less acute when an expected death occurs, but it is, nonetheless, invariably present.

Yearning. A longing for the return of the deceased. Feelings of loss, sorrow, and regret combine to pack an emotional punch, often accompanied by an actual physical aching.

Disorganization and despair. A feeling that life has lost its meaning, that one's very existence has been shaken by the experience of the loss.

Reorganization. Survivors put the pieces of their lives back together in such a way as to accommodate their loss.

How do you know when your mourning has been successful?

- First, you haven't denied either the loss or its impact on you. You've allowed yourself to acknowledge the full extent of your pain.

- Second, you've worked through your feelings by expressing and experiencing them.

- Third, you've adjusted to an environment from which the person is absent. No longer do you expect to encounter the person you have lost. "Sightings" of the deceased by survivors, often reported during the first few months after a loss—especially a traumatic one—have come to an end. You have come to terms with the fact that life will go on, though it will be different. One woman, reflecting upon coming to terms with her mother's death, said, "When I think of my mother, I remember how fortunate I was. I don't miss my mother anymore. I remember her."

When Grief Continues

There is no such thing as abnormal grieving. However, when grief continues indefinitely, and feelings of pain and distress linger, you may need help in order to come to terms with the death. Use the following list to clarify whether you have come to terms with your loss. Check each item that is true for you.

Are You Still Grieving?

_____ 1. Your intense sadness hasn't lightened even though many months have passed since the death.

_____ 2. You still feel responsible in some way for the death. (This is especially likely if the death was one of the types we described earlier as difficult to accept. It is especially true of suicide.)

_____ 3. You cry uncontrollably when you see photos of the dead person or on anniversaries, holidays, and other occasions that cause you to remember him.

____ 4. You still have trouble concentrating on your job, getting along with co-workers, or completing your assigned tasks.

____ 5. You are relying on alcohol, over-the-counter medications, or illegal drugs to help you sleep or to make it through the day.

____ 6. You are having difficulties in your intimate relationships. Your partner may complain that you are angry, emotionally withdrawn, or remote.

____ 7. You are experiencing significant weight loss or gain.

____ 8. You have trouble sleeping, either by falling asleep at inappropriate times or by waking during the night.

____ 9. You avoid thinking and talking about the death.

Scoring: If you check only one or two of the items, you are probably recovering; if you check more than three or four, and it has been more than six months since the death, you may need some help to come to terms with your loss.

If you are still struggling with the death of your care recipient, make a special effort to talk with friends or family. A pastor, rabbi, or other trained professional may also be of help. You need to find an emotionally safe environment, such as a bereavement support group, in which to work through your grief and move on with your life. In the following chapter, we discuss the function that support groups can serve in coping with caregiving and its aftermath.

CHAPTER TWELVE

CAREGIVER SUPPORT GROUPS

Over the past several years caregiver support groups have proliferated, varying widely along many dimensions, such as number of participants, purpose, makeup, and dynamics. In this chapter, we provide general information about them. We also guide you through the maze of such groups, help you to decide whether support groups are for you, point out the factors to consider when choosing one, and offer advice on forming your own.

Throughout this book, we have alluded to caregivers who could profit from the advice and emotional support of others. If you are such a person, one of the best ways to meet these needs is by joining a group made up of other caregivers, who share experiences and concerns similar to your own.

Why Are Caregiver Support Groups Popular?

Although caregiver support groups vary widely in type and quality, they all provide a place where people with common experiences and problems can give emotional support to one another, share information, and learn skills. Sometimes, after group members get to know each other and form friendships, they offer more tangible help, such as providing respite services (time off) when needed. For example, after we had led one group for several weeks, members began exchanging phone numbers and arranging to help each other out.

If a support group is well run, most people benefit. Said one woman who had participated in an effective group, "I got more out of this group during my mother's illness than I got from the therapist I was seeing. These people knew where I was coming from. Their help was delivered simply, without jargon, and they really cared."

Another participant observed, "Being part of the group helped me to learn how to take care of myself while still helping my husband. I learned to share responsibilities with other family members. Maybe most important, I learned that it was OK to ask for help, and to accept it when it was offered."

A third support group member commented that the group had afforded her the opportunity to express feelings. "There was really no one else I could talk to about the stress I was under. I was so exhausted most of the time. To have complained to my husband would have served no purpose—except to make him even more annoyed with me. The group provided an outlet for me that I would not have had otherwise."

Anecdotal evidence like this indicates that such groups clearly meet people's needs. However, not all groups are well run or contain a compatible mix of people, and variables such as these ultimately determine how helpful the group will be for its members.

What Should You Look For in a Support Group?

Based on our experiences as group leaders and participants, we have identified seven key factors you should consider when selecting a support group. They are as follows:

1. *Look for a group led by a person with professional credentials.* Many support groups are not led by professionals. Although having a leader trained in group behavior is no guarantee that the group will be properly led, lay people, even experienced caregivers, may not possess the skills and insights that make them effective group leaders. In fact, some caregivers may be too personally invested in their own problems to lead a group successfully.

   Unlike Alcoholics Anonymous and similar groups with long histories and clearly delineated procedures, caregiver support groups are rather new. There are few guidelines for leaders, leaving much up to the individual in charge. That person's skill and training can make the difference between a positive or a negative group experience.

2. *Look for a group with a leader who has been a caregiver, or is one.* A leader with caregiving experience has firsthand knowledge of what group members are going through and is more likely to be empathic and understanding.

3. *Look for a group that has been in existence for some time.* If the group you are considering is ongoing, look for one that has some longevity. Ineffective groups often dissolve because members stop attending and do not recommend the group to others. By contrast, well-run groups constantly attract new members.

4. *Look for a group with clear goals.* The group you join should have a clear overall focus. Moreover, each meeting should have a specific purpose. For example, in our groups, at times we ask members to discuss their own difficulties and to be prepared to troubleshoot for each other. At other times, we focus on feelings or arrange for guest speakers (physicians, attorneys, and others) to share information with the group. Regardless of what the purpose is, there always is one.

5. *Understand who the group is for.* Some groups are general in nature. They cater to the needs of all caregivers—whether they are caring for an aging relative or a spouse with cancer. Others are tied to a specific disability or condition, such as cancer or multiple sclerosis. There are benefits to both general groups and specifically focused ones. Whichever type you choose, be attentive to the makeup of the group and the quality of leadership.

6. *Understand that a support group is not intended to provide psychotherapy for its members.* The goals of these groups are to provide support for issues affecting caregivers. Generally, it is not appropriate to focus on issues that are more personal in nature. Although members are not usually screened for psychological problems, a skilled leader will recognize those individuals who are in need of more intensive help and refer them for appropriate treatment. At the very least, they should not be allowed to take over the group.

7. *Be aware of the unique features of the group.* In selecting a group, consider whether the plan for the group suits you. Here are some of the ways groups differ:

- Some groups are time-limited. You may be told at the beginning that the group will meet for a predetermined number of sessions, each lasting a certain amount of time. The goal of this type of experience is likely to be very limited, and the agenda for each session will almost certainly be spelled out. For example, we recently received a flyer announcing a four-session training program—described as a "caregiver course"—for caregivers whose care recipients have Alzheimer's disease. The goal of the group was to enhance both the knowledge and skills of family members, friends, and hired caregivers. The program was described as free and open to the public, and consisted primarily of presentations by physicians, nurses, social workers, and occupational therapists.

- Other groups are open-ended, less formal, and more cathartic in focus. Members are invited to share their problems and can look forward to the emotional support of others. These groups have a more general focus, and are more likely to be ongoing.

- In some groups, especially emotion-focused ones, membership may close once the group has begun in order to allow members to form ties. Other groups, especially those that are informational in nature, may allow anyone to join at any time.

- Groups also vary by how often they meet—weekly, biweekly, or monthly. Your needs and schedule will determine your preference in this regard.

How Can You Judge the Effectiveness of a Group?

When you join a support group, you are making an investment of time and energy. Because it is seldom convenient to make the arrangements necessary to attend, you want to be sure that the group is working for you.

One way to do this is to trust your feelings. Do you enjoy attending sessions and do you get something out of them? Or do you leave feeling more upset and aggravated than when you arrived? When you share feelings in the group, are they accepted, or do you feel embarrassed or silly afterward? How comfortable is it to express negative feelings? If such feelings are judged harshly by the leader or other members, or if you are made to feel guilty, weird, or "bad" for having expressed negative feelings, find another group.

Another way to know whether the group is right for you is to observe what happens, or fails to happen, in the group. Does the leader stay in control? If the group meanders in every direction and if nothing useful comes out of the session, something is wrong. No member should be allowed to dominate the group or monopolize the time. A competent leader will exert enough control to give everyone a fair opportunity to speak, but not so much control that people feel intimidated.

After a reasonable time in the group, you should find that your coping skills are improved. Perhaps you realize, without thinking much about it, that you have learned specific skills that are helpful in managing your caregiving responsibilities. Perhaps an idea you encountered in your group offers you solace when you are stressed or feeling at your wit's end. These are indications that the investment you are making is paying off.

Where to Find Support Groups in Your Community

Often, caregivers learn about support groups informally, in conversations with other caregivers or during a chance meeting in a doctor's office. But not all are so lucky. If you know of no groups, we suggest you begin your exploration by trying the following sources of information and guidance: (1) Some states have a toll-free number that serves as a clearing house for many services. Other states provide no single number. However, your phone directory may list numbers that can point you in the right direction. Since the investment in time and effort is small, this is a good place to start. (2) Your care recipient's physician, or a member of her/his office staff, may know of a group. (3) Your local hospital likely has a community relations office. Many such offices are kept up-to-date on local groups. (4) Organizations such as the Alzheimer's Association and Cancer Care often sponsor groups that are tied to these specific disorders. See the Resources section in the back of this book. We provide the phone numbers and addresses of such organizations, as well as for agencies that can help you locate support groups. (5) The Internet can be a useful source of information—about on-line caregiver support groups (not as good as an *in-person* group, but better than nothing), and about groups in different communities.

Are Support Groups for You?

Support groups are not for everyone. One reason they are not is that it is assumed group members will share their problems, worries, and concerns. If you are not willing to do that, a support group may not be comfortable for you. On the other hand, if your needs are so urgent that you *must* speak at length at every meeting or you need a great deal of attention, an individual meeting with a pastor, rabbi, good friend, or a therapist may be more useful to you.

Forming Your Own Caregiver Support Group

If you are unable to locate a caregiver support group, you may want to start one. Although doing this requires considerable time and effort, you may help yourself and others by doing so. Here are the steps to follow.

Before doing anything, think carefully about the group you want to launch. For whom is the group designed? What will its goals be? (We suggest that you answer the kinds of questions listed earlier in this chapter, but from the point of view of the person creating the group.) Once you have a clear idea of the group's purpose and have anticipated most of the questions likely to be asked by prospective members and group leaders, set your ideas down on paper and begin making contact with others.

Approach local professionals who may have an interest in caregiving and may be willing to lead a group. A letter or a few phone calls to psychotherapists or physicians may elicit responses from interested people. Explain what you have in mind and assess their interest in leading such a group. Tactfully check credentials. Discuss the commitment you would expect from the leader. Make clear whether the leader would earn any fees. Most groups charge no fee to members. As a rule, leaders donate their time—sometimes out of pure altruism, sometimes in an effort to build their practices, and sometimes both.

Locate prospective members by preparing a notice or flyer and hand-deliver or send copies of it to hospital admissions' offices, physicians' offices, merchants who sell home health-care supplies, pharmacies, and senior centers. The flyer should announce an organizational meeting. It should answer the following questions:

- Who is the group for?
- Where and when will the meeting take place?
- How long will it last?
- Will there be a fee?

Provide other relevant information such as directions to the meeting location. Two sample notices of organizational meeting announcements we used not long ago are on this page and page 168. Use them as models to create your own flyer.

Support Group for Caregivers of the Elderly

On [specific day] at [specific time] a meeting of people who provide care for an elderly relative or friend will take place at [specific location] to launch a caregiver support group.

Nature of Group: This is a professionally led support group for individuals who provide care for seniors. Family, friends, spouses, and others are all welcome. Group will meet weekly and will be ongoing, with no specific end date in mind. Membership will change during the group's life, with some members leaving and others joining at various points.

Purposes of Group: The group will be a vehicle for mutual support and problem solving, as well as for education and learning specific skills.

Location, Length, and Time of Meetings: The group will meet every Thursday from 7:30 to 9:00 P.M. at a location to be determined. (Size of group will determine location of meetings. Some possibilities: our town's Senior Center, a private therapist's office, a local nursing home, or an adult day-care center.)

Fees: There are no fees for attendance.

Directions to Meeting Site: [give directions]
Coffee and snacks will be provided

Here is an alternate format for your flyer:

A Support Group for Caregivers of the Elderly

Nature of Group: This is a support group for individuals who provide care for seniors. Family, friends, spouses, and others are all welcome. Group will be ongoing, with no specific end date in mind. Membership will change during the group's life, with some members leaving and others joining at various points.

Purposes of Group: The group will be a vehicle for mutual support and problem solving, as well as for education and learning specific skills such as assertive communication.

Location, Length, and Time of Meetings: The group will meet at a time agreed upon by members, for 90 minutes, at a place suitable for the conduct of the group's business. (See below for location of organizational meeting.)

Organizational Meeting: Interested people should plan to attend an hour-long organizational meeting, to be held at [specific location], on [specific date], at [specific time]. Directions: Route XX to shopping center [etc.] Please call [phone number] to confirm your intention to attend and for additional information.

Fees: There are no fees for attendance. However, a $5.00 per person or per couple room rental fee is requested. Once a non-fee location is found for regular meetings, no fees of any sort will be requested.

Leader: The organizational meeting will be led by [name and credentials of leader].

Use the flyer you prepare as the basis for an ad in your local paper. Ask the community relations editor to run a press release or perhaps arrange for an interview. Here is an example of a press release to guide you:

Support Group for Caregivers of the Elderly

Local residents providing care for an elderly relative or friend are invited to a free, hour-long meeting to be held on [specific date], at [specific time], in [specific location].

The purpose of the meeting is to discuss the formation of a caregiver support group. The planned group will be professionally led by [name and credentials of leader], and will have as its goals to enhance the caregiving skills of members while providing emotional support.

Pre-registration is required. Please call 555-5555. All registrations will be acknowledged.

At the organizational meeting assess the attendees' interest in launching a group. Review the group's purposes and design. Encourage questions, and afterwards obtain the necessary information for those questions you cannot answer. Discuss the commitment expected of those who join the group. Allow the leader you have designated to introduce himself or herself. Together, all attendees should decide on the time and place of the next meeting.

A Final Word

Many caregivers feel they cannot afford the time to attend support groups. "If I could get out once a week or once a month to attend a support group meeting," said one man, "I wouldn't need one!" Such reasoning may seem persuasive, but it is just another way to avoid self-care. Effective caregiving requires a great deal of the caregiver—specific skills, emotional resilience, and creativity—and any source of support should be welcomed. Ultimately, not only will you benefit from a well-run caregiver support group, but your caregiving will be enhanced as well.

EXERCISES AND ACTIVITIES FOR DUPLICATION AND USE IN SUPPORT GROUPS

This Appendix consists of exercises, activities, worksheets, and checklists that appear in earlier chapters. They are grouped here for your convenience and are in the same order in which they appear throughout the book. If you would rather not write in the book, you can photocopy anything from this Appendix and then write on the pages you reproduced. You have our permission to duplicate all materials, but we ask you to be sure that the credit that appears at the end of each activity be included in the copies you duplicate, especially if you distribute them to others. (This represents no effort on your part. All you need do is ensure that the entire page is photo-copied.)

All of these activities are recommended for use in caregiver support groups. (See chapter 12 for information about support groups.)

A Note to Caregiver Support Group Facilitators

Here are some suggestions for how to use the activities that follow:

1. The first three can help "break the ice" and encourage group members to get to know one another by comparing their experiences. Why did they become caregivers? How do their caregiving functions differ? How are they similar? Group members can also help you create a group profile that can be used to show the extent to which they are typical or atypical caregivers. This can be an interesting activity, while serving to inform or remind your members that their caregiving experience—or some variation on it—is shared by literally millions of individuals across the country.

2. Other activities can help members solve problems. Activity Four (The Terms of an Informal Interpersonal Contract) and Activity Five (Caregiver Checklist: Who's in Control) can help to clarify whose needs predominate in the caregiving relationship. Activity Six (Caregiving Contract Worksheet) can help to implement needed changes.

   Similarly, Activities Seven (Warning Signs of Caregiver Burnout) and Nine (Preventing Burnout) can help alert the caregiver who may be at risk. Activities Ten (Resistance to Self-Care) and Eleven (Caregiver's Logsheet) can avert the problem.

3. Some activities are excellent starting points for discussion of various issues. For example, Activity Eight (The Caregiver's Bill of Rights) will encourage discussion among members about their rights as caregivers. You may also want to have members modify or add to the rights that are listed.

4. Activity Twelve, Parts One through Four, are logsheets, intended to help caregivers record and organize important information. Members may wish to share techniques that they have found helpful. Often, just discussing record-keeping is enormously helpful to people who feel over-whelmed by the complexities of doing battle with insurance company personnel.

5. Some activities, such as Thirteen (Were You a Reverse Role Caregiver?), can be used by members to help them under-stand why they may have assumed their current caregiving roles.

We invite you to use these activities in whatever ways make the most sense. We welcome your comments and suggestions. Please write to us c/o New Harbinger Publications, 5674 Shattuck Avenue, Oakland, California, 94609.

Activity One: Your Caregiver Profile

Directions: Please answer each of the following questions by checking the appropriate box.

1. Your sex:
   - ☐ M
   - ☐ F

2. Your age:
   - ☐ Under 30
   - ☐ 30–39
   - ☐ 40–49
   - ☐ 50–59
   - ☐ 60 or above

3. Your relationships:
   - ☐ Married or live with partner
   - ☐ Single, divorced, separated, or widowed

4. Your responsibilities in addition to caregiving:
   - ☐ Work inside the home
     - ☐ homemaking
     - ☐ home-based business
     - ☐ care for children under age 18
     - ☐ care for children over age 18
   - ☐ Work outside the home
     - ☐ parttime employment
     - ☐ fulltime employment

5. Percent of caregiving responsibilities that fall on you:
   - ☐ 100 % (you are the sole caregiver)
   - ☐ You share caregiving responsibilities with others
     - ☐ bulk (more than 50%) of caregiving responsibilities fall on you
     - ☐ bulk of caregiving responsibilities fall on one or more other persons

6. The person for whom you provide care:

- □ spouse or partner
- □ child
- □ parent
- □ sibling, friend, relative, or other

Copied with permission from Ilardo and Rothman, *I'll Take Care of You: A Practical Guide for Family Caregivers.* Oakland, CA: New Harbinger Publications, 1999. To order the book, call 800-748-6273.

Activity Two: The Caregiving Services You Provide

Directions: Please put a checkmark on the appropriate lines.

1. As a caregiver, I primarily:

   ____ Provide companionship and show concern through calls and occasional visits

   ____ Take my care recipient to lunch

   ____ Shop with my care recipient

   ____ Arrange for occasional outings

2. As a caregiver, I primarily:

   ____ Arrange medical appointments, coordinate schedules, etc.

   ____ Take my care recipient to medical appointments; provide transport for laboratory tests, and take him/her to and from procedures (such as surgeries) performed on an outpatient basis

   ____ Consult with members of my care recipient's health care team and make decisions in consultation with my care recipient

   ____ Shop for my care recipient

   ____ Prepare some meals for my care recipient

3. As a caregiver, I primarily:

   ____ Provide homemaking services (do laundry, clean house, etc.)

   ____ Arrange for home repairs, maintenance, etc.

   ____ Prepare most or all meals

   ____ Arrange for care when I can't be there

   ____ Pay bills

4. As a caregiver, I primarily:

   ____ Provide help with bathing, dressing, eating, and using the toilet

   ____ Assist with the management of incontinence

   ____ Help my care recipient cope despite serious cognitive disabilities (for example, the forgetfulness and lack of orientation characteristic of Alzheimer's disease)

   ____ Arrange for home-health aides and others to provide help when I am not available

5. As a caregiver, I primarily:

_____ Help my care recipient prepare advance directives such as a living will

_____ Serve as health care proxy

_____ Serve as attorney-in-fact for most or all other matters; manage all financial affairs, etc.

Copied with permission from Ilardo and Rothman, *I'll Take Care of You: A Practical Guide for Family Caregivers*. Oakland, CA: New Harbinger Publications, 1999. To order the book, call 800-748-6273.

Activity Three, Part One: Why You Became a Caregiver

Directions: Please indicate the extent to which, in your opinion, each factor resulted in your becoming a caregiver. Mark each scale at the appropriate point.

1. **Social Expectations**

   I have become a caregiver because of

   a. my sex

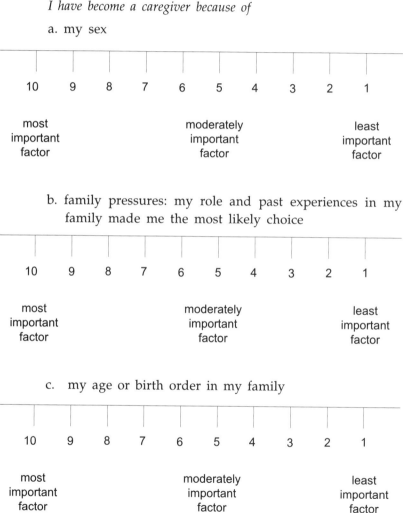

| 10 | 9 | 8 | 7 | 6 | 5 | 4 | 3 | 2 | 1 |

most
important
factor

moderately
important
factor

least
important
factor

   b. family pressures: my role and past experiences in my family made me the most likely choice

| 10 | 9 | 8 | 7 | 6 | 5 | 4 | 3 | 2 | 1 |

most
important
factor

moderately
important
factor

least
important
factor

   c. my age or birth order in my family

| 10 | 9 | 8 | 7 | 6 | 5 | 4 | 3 | 2 | 1 |

most
important
factor

moderately
important
factor

least
important
factor

I have become a caregiver because of

d. I live with or nearest to the care recipient

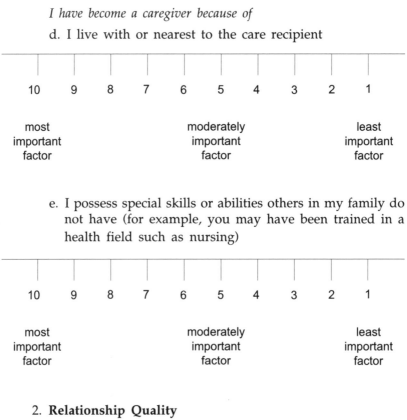

e. I possess special skills or abilities others in my family do not have (for example, you may have been trained in a health field such as nursing)

2. Relationship Quality

I have become a caregiver because of

my especially close relationship with the care recipient

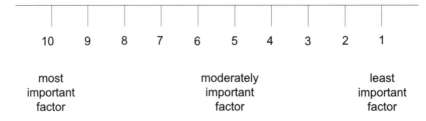

3. **Self-Perceptions**

I have become a caregiver because of

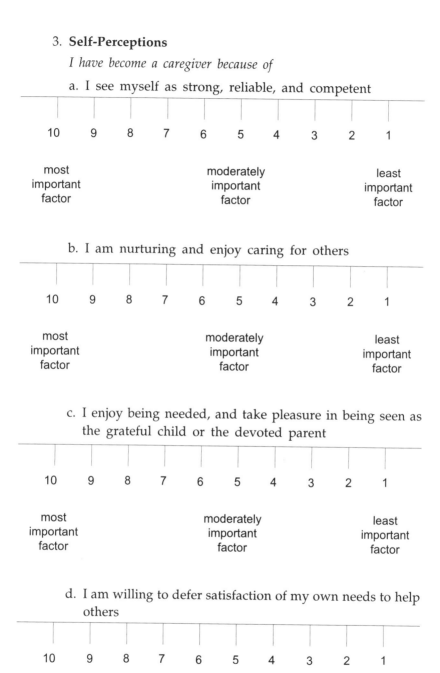

a. I see myself as strong, reliable, and competent

| 10 | 9 | 8 | 7 | 6 | 5 | 4 | 3 | 2 | 1 |

most
important
factor

moderately
important
factor

least
important
factor

b. I am nurturing and enjoy caring for others

| 10 | 9 | 8 | 7 | 6 | 5 | 4 | 3 | 2 | 1 |

most
important
factor

moderately
important
factor

least
important
factor

c. I enjoy being needed, and take pleasure in being seen as the grateful child or the devoted parent

| 10 | 9 | 8 | 7 | 6 | 5 | 4 | 3 | 2 | 1 |

most
important
factor

moderately
important
factor

least
important
factor

d. I am willing to defer satisfaction of my own needs to help others

| 10 | 9 | 8 | 7 | 6 | 5 | 4 | 3 | 2 | 1 |

most
important
factor

moderately
important
factor

least
important
factor

4. Accident and Circumstances

I have become a caregiver because of

illness, accident, or other circumstances beyond my control

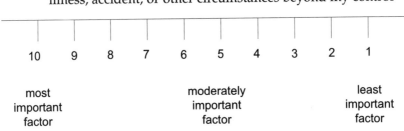

| 10 | 9 | 8 | 7 | 6 | 5 | 4 | 3 | 2 | 1 |

most
important
factor

moderately
important
factor

least
important
factor

Activity Three, Part Two: Why You Became a Caregiver

Directions: Each item in Column A corresponds to each question you just completed. In Column B, record the numeric score you marked above. Then plot the numbers on the grid that appears at the bottom of this exercise.

Column A

Factor

Column B

Score You Earned
(10 = most important,
1 = least)

1. Social Expectations

Sex _____

Family pressures: roles and past experiences in the family _____

Age or birth order _____

Physical proximity to care recipient _____

Special skills and abilities _____

2. Relationship Quality (emotional closeness to care recipient) _____

3. Self-Perceptions _____

See myself as strong, reliable, and competent _____

Nurturing personality _____

Enjoy being needed _____

Willing to defer personal satisfaction _____

4. Accident and Circumstances _____

Now plot on the grid below the number score you wrote on each line:

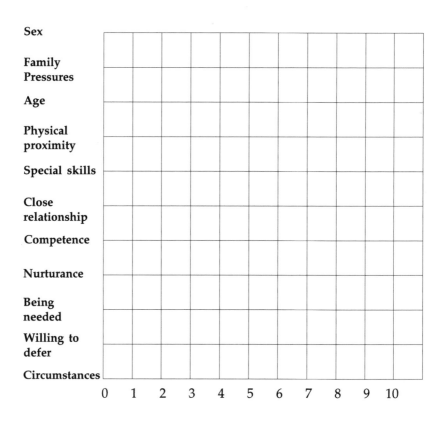

Sex

Family
Pressures

Age

Physical
proximity

Special skills

Close
relationship

Competence

Nurturance

Being
needed

Willing to
defer

Circumstances

0   1   2   3   4   5   6   7   8   9   10

Copied with permission from Ilardo and Rothman, *I'll Take Care of You: A Practical Guide for Family Caregivers.* Oakland, CA: New Harbinger Publications, 1999. To order the book, call 800-748-6273.

Activity Four: The Terms of an Informal Interpersonal Contract

Directions: In this exercise you are asked to uncover the contractual basis for one of your close relationships. For the purposes of this activity, you should write about someone other than your care recipient. Please use the spaces provided to write about your expectations, rights and responsibilities, as well as those of the person with whom you have a close relationship.

Expectations

1. Things I expect of my relationship partner (for example, you might expect a good friend to remember your birthday, your sibling to feed your cats when you go away, or your spouse to schedule vacations to coincide with your time off work).

_____

_____

_____

2. Things my relationship partner expects of me (for example, a good friend might expect you to remember her birthday, a younger sibling might expect you to help with homework, and your spouse might expect you to take out the garbage).

_____

_____

_____

Rights

1. My rights (for example, you have the right to get off the phone with your friend if you don't feel like talking any longer).

_____

_____

_____

2. My relationship partner's rights (for example, your sibling may have the right to ask you to lower the volume on your CD player).

_____

_____

_____

Responsibilities

1. My responsibilities (for example, you might feel obligated to do your share around the house).

_____

_____

_____

2. My relationship partner's responsibilities (for example, your spouse may be in charge of changing the oil in the family car).

_____

_____

_____

Activity Five: Caregiver Checklist: Who's in Control?

Directions: Please respond to each of the questions below by circling Y for *yes* or N for *no*.

1. Within the past week, I found myself re-arranging my schedule on short notice to meet nonessential needs of my care recipient. Y N

2. When I think carefully about events that have transpired over the last several months, I realize that my care recipient's crises have coincided with important events in my life or my family's. Y N

3. Even though my care recipient is not critically ill, I sometimes put off doing things I would enjoy (going to dinner with a friend, for example) because he may need me. Y N

4. I feel so sorry for my care recipient that I feel guilty enjoying anything. Y N

5. It seems the harder I work to provide loving care, the more my care recipient expects of me. Y N

6. If I am unavailable, my care recipient creates crises to force others to take care of him. Y N

7. No matter what the doctor says, my superior and consistent care will make my recipient better. Y N

8. Sometimes my care recipient doesn't do what he is told, or fails to make an honest effort to help himself. Y N

9. When my care recipient feels anxious or depressed, I find myself feeling that way, too. Y N

10. I sometimes refuse offers of help because I am convinced no one else can provide the same level and quality of care that I provide. Y N

Scoring: Give yourself one point for every Y you circled. If you scored 5 or above on the quiz, it's likely that dependency and control conflicts are adversely affecting your relationship with your care recipient.

Copied with permission from Ilardo and Rothman, *I'll Take Care of You: A Practical Guide for Family Caregivers.* Oakland, CA: New Harbinger Publications, 1999. To order the book, call 800-748-6273.

Activity Six: Caregiving Contract Worksheet

Directions: You and your care recipient should cooperate in responding to the following items.

I. Caregiver's Rights

As the caregiver in this relationship, I now have the following rights (for example, the right to take coffee breaks):

1. _____

2. _____

3. _____

As the caregiver in this relationship, I wish to add the following rights:

1. _____

2. _____

3. _____

II. Caregiver's Responsibilities

As the caregiver in this relationship, I now have the following responsibilities (for example, administering a daily sponge bath):

1. _____

2. _____

3. _____

As the caregiver in this relationship, I wish to alter my responsibilities as follows:

1. _____

2. _____

3. _____

III. Care Recipient's Rights

The care recipient in this relationship now has the following rights (for example, the right to request help at any time).

1. _____

2. _____

3. _____

The care recipient's rights will be expanded or limited as follows:

1. _____

2. _____

3. _____

IV. Care Recipient's Responsibilities

The care recipient in this relationship now has the following responsibilities (for example, he is responsible for dressing himself in the morning).

1. _____

2. _____

3. _____

The care recipient's responsibilities will be expanded or limited as follows:

1. _____

2. _____

3. _____

Copied with permission from Ilardo and Rothman, *I'll Take Care of You: A Practical Guide for Family Caregivers*. Oakland, CA: New Harbinger Publications, 1999. To order the book, call 800-748-6273.

Activity Seven: Warning Signs of Caregiver Burnout

Directions: Please respond to each item by circling Y for *yes* or N for *no.*

1. I feel sad and "down" more often than is usual for me.   Y   N
2. Lately, I am doing fewer and fewer of the things I enjoy.   Y   N
3. I often feel overwhelmed and pressured.   Y   N
4. I feel very alone much of the time.   Y   N
5. I often cry.   Y   N
6. I prefer not to talk about my stresses or problems with others.   Y   N
7. I sometimes fear my anger will get out of control.   Y   N
8. I react strongly to little annoyances.   Y   N
9. I'm afraid I'll do something to injure my care recipient.   Y   N
10. I resent it when other people have a good time.   Y   N
11. I feel "edgy" much of the time.   Y   N
12. I often feel something terrible is about to happen.   Y   N

Activity Eight: Caregiver's Bill of Rights

As a caregiver, I have the right . . .

- To take care of myself—to rest when I'm tired, to eat well, to take breaks from caregiving when I need to
- To recognize the limits of my own endurance and strength
- To seek help from family, involved parties, and the community at large
- To socialize, to maintain my interests, and to do things I enjoy
- To acknowledge my feelings, whether positive or negative, including frustration, anger, and depression, and to express them constructively
- To take pride in the valuable work I do, and to applaud the courage and inventiveness it takes to meet the needs of my care recipient

Copied with permission from Ilardo and Rothman, *I'll Take Care of You: A Practical Guide for Family Caregivers*. Oakland, CA: New Harbinger Publications, 1999. To order the book, call 800-748-6273.

Activity Nine: Preventing Burnout

Directions: Review your answers to the items in the inventory you completed earlier . If you responded to an item affirmatively (by circling Y), carefully consider each set of questions that follows the statement below, then use the space provided to formulate your action plan. As you do so, be sure to consider exactly what you plan to do, when, and how.

1. I feel sad and "down" more often than is normal for me.   Y   N

   Questions to ask yourself: When do I feel better? Does anything cause my "down" mood to lift? For example, does a change in my daily routine help? Is my sadness related to anything I can control ? Do I get sad when I feel taken advantage of by others? If so, what can I do to help myself?

   My Plan: I will schedule a mid-morning "newspaper and coffee" break, starting tomorrow.

2. Lately, I am doing fewer of the things I enjoy.   Y   N

   Questions to ask yourself: Within the next few days, what would I enjoy doing? Is there a movie I'd like to see? A restaurant I want to try? A TV show I'd like to watch?

   My Plan:

   _____

   _____

   _____

3. I often feel overwhelmed and pressured.   Y   N

   Questions to ask yourself: Where is this pressure coming from? What can I do to reduce it? Can I delegate responsibilities? Accept offers of help from others? Reduce my other commitments?

   My Plan:

   _____

   _____

   _____

4. I feel very alone much of the time.   Y   N

Questions to ask yourself: To whom might I talk? Can I call a friend? Is there someone, such as a rabbi or pastor, with whom I can share my distress?

My Plan:

_____

_____

_____

5. I often cry.   Y   N

Questions to ask yourself: What words are my tears expressing? How can I help myself feel better?

My Plan:

_____

_____

_____

6. I prefer not to talk about my stresses or problems with others.   Y   N

Questions to ask yourself: Who might I feel safe talking with? How can I contact them? What lay or professional helpers are available to me?

My Plan:

_____

_____

_____

7. I sometimes feel my anger will get out of control.   Y   N

Questions to ask yourself: When do I get angry? What can I do to direct that anger appropriately? Can I, for example, confront someone who is not doing his share?

My Plan:

_____

_____

_____

8. I react strongly to little annoyances.   Y   N

Questions to ask yourself: Why am I reacting as I am? What do these strong reactions suggest? Where should my annoyance really be directed?

My Plan:

_____

_____

_____

9. I'm afraid I'll do something to injure my care recipient.   Y   N

Questions to ask yourself: What am I angry about? Who can help me sort out my feelings? How can I come to grips with my anger and resentment? Could I benefit from speaking to a mental health specialist?

My Plan:

_____

_____

_____

10. I resent it when other people have a good time.   Y   N

Questions to ask yourself: What is causing me to feel this resentment? What positive steps can I take that would make my everyday life more pleasant?

My Plan:

_____

_____

_____

11. I feel "edgy" much of the time. Y N

Questions to ask yourself: What is causing this "edgy" feeling? Am I giving myself time to unwind? Am I relying on caffeine or other substances to enable me to keep going when I really need to rest?

My Plan:

_____

_____

_____

12. I often feel something terrible is about to happen. Y N

Questions to ask yourself: Since this is a symptom of anxiety, what steps can I take on my own to reduce my anxiety level? Could I benefit from a stress management group? Should I see a mental health profession to help me manage my anxiety?

My Plan:

_____

_____

_____

Copied with permission from Ilardo and Rothman, *I'll Take Care of You: A Practical Guide for Family Caregivers.* Oakland, CA: New Harbinger Publications, 1999. To order the book, call 800-748-6273.

Activity Ten: Resistance to Self-Care

Directions: We have listed below the reasons caregivers typically give for avoiding self-care. Take a moment to read each of them, then formulate an argument to rebut it.

Reason One: "It's not I who needs care! I'm the healthy one!"

Your Rebuttal: _____

_____

_____

_____

Reason Two: "It's selfish. I can't do that to my care recipient."

Your Rebuttal: _____

_____

_____

_____

Reason Three: "Others will think I'm irresponsible."

Your Rebuttal: _____

_____

_____

_____

Reason Four: "I'd never forgive myself if something happened while I was out having a good time!"

Your Rebuttal: _____

_____

_____

_____

Reason Five: "I shouldn't need to take a break. I'm strong."

Your Rebuttal:

_____

_____

_____

Activity Eleven: Caregiver's Log Sheet

Caregiver's Logsheet

Date	How I Felt Before	What I Did	How I Felt After	When Will I Do It Again?	Remarks

Copied with permission from Ilardo and Rothman, *I'll Take Care of You: A Practical Guide for Family Caregivers*. Oakland, CA: New Harbinger Publications, 1999. To order the book, call 800-748-6273.

Activity Twelve, Part One: Log Sheets

Log Sheet: Letters Received

Date	Item Received	From Whom	Content of Message	Other

Activity Twelve, Part Two: Log Sheets

Log Sheet: Letters Sent

Date	Item Sent	To Whom	Content of Message	Other

Copied with permission from Ilardo and Rothman, *I'll Take Care of You: A Practical Guide for Family Caregivers.* Oakland, CA: New Harbinger Publications, 1999. To order the book, call 800-748-6273.

Activity Twelve, Part Three: Log Sheets

Log Sheet: Telephone Calls Received

Date	Who Called	Caller's number	Content of Message	Other

Activity Twelve, Part Four: Log Sheets

Log Sheet: Telephone Calls Placed

Date	Person Called	Their number	Content of Message	Other

Copied with permission from Ilardo and Rothman, *I'll Take Care of You: A Practical Guide for Family Caregivers.* Oakland, CA: New Harbinger Publications, 1999. To order the book, call 800-748-6273.

Activity Thirteen: Were You a Reverse Role Caregiver?

Directions: Please respond to each of the following statements by circling Y for *yes* and N for *no*.

1. If my parent was sad or upset, I felt I had to cheer him/her up.
   Y   N

2. I was often made to feel guilty if I chose to be with friends instead of with my parent.   Y   N

3. My parent sometimes asked me to sleep in his/her bed for company.   Y   N

4. When my parent hugged me, I often felt as if I wanted to break free and run.   Y   N

5. I sometimes felt I was my parent's partner rather than his/her child.   Y   N

6. When things went wrong at home, my parent(s) looked to me to make things better.   Y   N

7. I often lent money to my parent.   Y   N

8. I was usually expected to take care of my siblings because my parents were unable to do so.   Y   N

9. I often wished my parents had a better relationship so I would be off the hook.   Y   N

10. I was often asked to side with one parent against the other.
    Y   N

Authorization to Release and Exchange Information

I (print name) _____ residing at
(print address and phone number) _____
_____ hereby authorize _____
(name of therapist) to release information about my treatment with
the following individual: _____
(print your name and your relationship with the care recipient).

I understand that by signing this form, I am agreeing to hold
_____ (name of therapist) harmless
with respect to any and all uses to which the information he/she
releases with my authorization are put.

This authorization expires on _____ .

Signed _____ Date _____

Witness _____(waived)_____ Date _____

RESOURCES

These resources have been selected for excellence as well as for ease of use. They are organized by category. Within each category, as available, we have listed publications, organizations, hotlines, and websites. Each website listed can serve as a point of entry to many related sites.

Death and Suicide

Publications

Humphrey, Derek. 1992. *Dying with Dignity*. New York: Carol Communications.

Kübler-Ross, Elisabeth. 1981. *Living with Death and Dying*. New York: Collier Books.

———. 1969. *On Death and Dying*. New York: Macmillan.

Organizations

American Association of Suicidology
4201 Connecticut Avenue NW, Suite 310
Washington, DC 20008
202-237-2280

Americans for Better Care of the Dying
2175 K Street, NW, Suite 820
Washington, DC 20037-1803
202-530-9864

Choice in Dying
200 Varick Street
New York, NY 10014-4810
800-989-9455

Foundation for Hospice and Homecare
519 C Street NE
Washington, DC 20002
202-547-5263

Hotline

National Hospice Organization
800-658-8898

Disabilities and Chronic Conditions

Publications

The Complete Directory for People with Disabilities. 1998. Lakeville, CT:
Grey House Publishing.
Reilly, Richard L. 1993. *Living with Pain.* Minneapolis, MN: Deaconess
Press.

Organizations

There are hundreds of organizations devoted to helping people
with specific disabilities, for example, The Arthritis Foundation, 1314
Spring Street NW, Atlanta, GA 30309, 404-872-7682, and The
National Multiple Sclerosis Society, 733 Third Avenue, New York,
NY 10017, 212-986-3240. Your local librarian can direct you to the
organization that focuses specifically on the disability or chronic
condition from which your care recipient may suffer. Here we list
only representative organizations.

American Paralysis Association
500 Morris Avenue
Springfield, NJ 07081
800-225-0292

Hotlines

American Trauma Society
800-556-7890

Cancer Information Center
800-4-Cancer

National Institute of Neurological and Stroke Disorders
800-352-9424

Eldercare

Publications

Cohen, Donna, and Carl Eisendorfer. 1993. *Caring for Your Aging Parents*. New York: Putnam.

Federal Trade Commission and American Association of Retired Persons. Ten-part series of pamphlets on eldercare. Available from the Consumer Response Center at the FTC, 202-382-4357.
The series includes titles such as: *Consumer Fraud Against the Elderly* and *Long-Term Care Insurance*.

Feldesman, Walter. 1997. *Dictionary of Eldercare Terminology*. Washington, DC: United Seniors Health Cooperative.

Hayflick, Leonard. 1994. *How and Why We Age*. New York: Ballantine Books.

Heath, Angela. 1993. *Long-Distance Caregiving*. San Luis Obispo, CA: Impact Publishers.

Ilardo, Joseph. 1998. *As Parents Age: A Psychological and Practical Guide*. Acton, MA: VanderWyk & Burnham.

Loverde, Joy. 1997. *The Complete Elder Care Planner*. New York: Hyperion.

Lustbader, Wendy. 1991. *Counting on Kindness: The Dilemmas of Dependency*. New York: Free Press.

Mace, Nancy L., and Peter V. Rabins. 1991. *The 36-Hour Day*. New York: Warner Books.

Organizations

Alzheimer's Association
919 North Michigan Avenue
Chicago, IL 60611
312-335-8700

American Association of Retired Persons
601 E Street NW
Washington, DC 20049
202-434-2277

National Association of Area Agencies on Aging
1112 16th Street NW, Suite 100
Washington, DC 20036
202-296-8130

National Hospice Organization
1901 North Moore Street, Suite 901
Arlington, VA 22209
800-658-8898

Hotlines

Eldercare Locator
800-677-1116

Hospice Helpline
800-658-8898

Websites

htpp://www.seniornet.com

htpp://www.aarp.org (American Association of Retired Persons)

htpp://www.ama-assn.org (American Medical Association)

htpp://www.nih.gov (National Institutes of Health)

http://www.nih.gov/nia/ (National Institute on Aging)

General Caregiving

Publications

Brandt, Avrene L. 1998. *Caregiver's Reprieve: A Guide to Emotional Survival When You're Caring for Someone You Love.* San Luis Obispo, CA: Impact Publishers.

Capossela, Cappy, and Sheila Warnock. 1995. *Share the Care: How to Organize a Group to Care for Someone Who Is Seriously Ill.* New York: Fireside.

Carter, Rosalynn, with Susan Golant. 1994. *Helping Yourself Help Others.* New York: Random House.

Lustbader, Wendy. 1991. *Counting on Kindness: The Dilemmas of Dependency.* New York: The Free Press.

National Family Caregivers Association. 1996. *The Resourceful Caregiver: Helping Family Caregivers Help Themselves.* St. Louis Missouri: Mosby Yearbook, Inc.

Smith, Wesley J. 1994. *Getting the Best From Your Doctor: A Nuts and Bolts Guide to Consumer Health.* Washington, DC: Center for Study of Responsive Law.

Today's Caregiver: America's Magazine for Family and Professional Caregivers. Edited by Gary Barg. P.O. Box 21646, Ft. Lauderdale, FL 33335.

Organizations

Patients' Rights Hotline
215 West 125th Street
New York, NY 10027
212-316-9393

National Association for Home Care
519 C Street NE, Stanston Park
Washington, DC 20002
202-547-7424

National Caregiving Foundation
401 Wythe Street, Suite A-3
PO Box 264
Alexandria, VA 22314
703-299-9300

National Family Caregivers Association
10605 Concord Street, Suite 501
Kensington, MD 20895-2504
800-896-3650

National Health Information Center
US Department of Health and Human Services
PO Box 1133
Washington, DC 20013
800-336-4797

Hotlines

National Caregiving Foundation
800-930-1357

Websites

htpp://www.healthnet.com

htpp://www.nfcares.org

htpp://www.caregiver.com (*Today's Caregiver* Magazine)

Mental Illness

Publications

Adamec, Christine. 1996. *How to Live with a Mentally Ill Person: A Handbook of Day-to-Day Strategies.* New York: John Wiley.

Cormier, Sid. 1993. *Am I Normal? Your Personal Guide to Understanding Yourself and Others.* New York: Carroll & Graf.

Torrey, E. Fuller. 1995. *Surviving Schizophrenia: A Manual For Families, Consumers, and Providers,* 3rd ed. New York: Harper/Perennial.

Wyden, Peter. 1998. *Conquering Schizophrenia.* New York: Knopf.

Organizations

Professional Associations

American Psychiatric Association
1400 K Street NW
Washington, DC 20005
202-682-6220

American Psychological Association
750 First Street NE
Washington, DC 20002-4242
202-336-5500

National Association of Social Workers
750 First Street NE, Suite 7700
Washington, DC 20002
800-638-8799

Lay Organizations

National Alliance for the Mentally Ill
200 North Glebe Road, Suite 1015
Arlington, VA 22203
800-950-6264

National Mental Health Association
1021 Prince Street
Alexandria, VA 22314-7722
800-969-6642

Government Agencies

National Institute of Mental Health
8901 Wisconsin Avenue
Rockville, MD 20895
301-443-4513

Organizations with a Specific Focus

National Alliance for Research on Schizophrenia and Depression
60 Cutter Mill Road, Suite 404
Great Neck, NY 11021
516-829-0091

National Depressive and Manic Depressive Association
730 Franklin Street, Suite 501
Chicago, IL 60610
312-642-0049

National Foundation for Depressive Illness
PO Box 2257
New York, NY 10116
800-248-4344

Hotlines

National Institute of Mental Health
800-421-4211

National Alliance for the Mentally Ill
800-950-6264

Websites

www.mentalhealth.com

www.nimh.nih.gov

www.psychology.com

Special Needs Children

Publications

Frith, Terry. 1985. *Secrets Parents Should Know About Public Schools.* New York: Simon and Schuster.

Silver, Larry B. 1998. *The Misunderstood Child—Understanding and Coping with Your Child's Learning Disabilities,* 3rd ed. New York: Times Books.

Taylor, John F. 1997. *Helping Your Hyperactive/ADD Child,* revised 2d ed. Rocklin, CA: Prima Publishing.

Weiss, Elizabeth. 1989. *Mothers Talk About Learning Disabilities: Personal Feelings, Practical Advice.* New York: Prentice Hall.

Hotlines

Children and Adults with Attention Deficit Disorder
499 Northwest 10th Avenue, Suite 101
Plantation, FL 33317
800-233-4050

National Dyslexic Research Foundation
800-824-7323

Websites

www.ldonline.org (learning disabilities)

www.ldanatl.org (learning disabilities)

www.ld-add.com (learning disabilities)

REFERENCES

Brody, Jane. 1998. Trying to cope when a partner or a loved one is chronically depressed. *New York Times.* January 6, F-9.

Cohen, Herb. 1989. *You Can Negotiate Anything.* New York: Bantam Books.

Family and Work Institute. 1998. *Work and Family Life.* Jacksonville: IL.

Fisher, Ian. 1998. Families providing complex medical care, tubes and all. *New York Times,* June 7, 1, 30.

Goffman, Erving. 1959. *The Presentation of Self in Everyday Life.* Garden City, New York: Anchor Books.

Lustbader, Wendy. 1991. *Counting on Kindness: The Dilemmas of Dependency.* New York: The Free Press.

National Alliance for the Mentally Ill. 1999. Estimates of Mental Illness Prevalence. http://www.nami.org/update/updatev.htm

National Family Caregivers Association. 1998. A Profile of Caregiving. *Take Care* 7:1(Winter): 7–8.

Shellenbarger, Sue. 1994. Many firms ignore new law on family leave. *Wall Street Journal,* July 27, D-8.

———. 1997. We take better care of our elderly parents than most realize. *Wall Street Journal,* March 12, B1.

INDEX

More New
Harbinger Titles

LIVING WELL WITH A HIDDEN DISABILITY

Provides a wealth of resources for healthy living, including advice on navigating the health care system and suggestions for strengthening the body, mind, and soul.

Item HID $15.95

THE CHRONIC PAIN CONTROL WORKBOOK

A team of specialists in all areas of pain management detail the treatment strategies for managing and recovering from chronic pain.

Item PN2 $18.95

WINNING AGAINST RELAPSE

A structured program teaches you how to monitor symptoms and respond to them in a way that reduces or eliminates the possibility of relapse.

Item WIN $14.95

FIBROMYALGIA & CHRONIC MYOFASCIAL PAIN SYNDROME

This survival manual is the first comprehensive patient guide for managing these conditions. Readers learn how to identify trigger points, cope with chronic pain and sleep problems, and deal with the numbing effects of "fibrofog."

Item FMS $19.95

THE HEADACHE AND NECK PAIN WORKBOOK

Combines the latest research with proven alternative therapies to help sufferers of head and neck pain understand and master their condition.

Item NECK $14.95

LAST TOUCH
Preparing for a Parent's Death

In death as well as birth, information about what happens and how to help can reduce fear and pain.

Item LAST $11.95

Call **toll-free 1-800-748-6273** to order. Have your Visa or Mastercard number ready. Or send a check for the titles you want to New Harbinger Publications, 5674 Shattuck Avenue, Oakland, CA 94609. Include $3.80 for the first book and 75¢ for each additional book to cover shipping and handling. (California residents please include appropriate sales tax.) Allow four to six weeks for delivery.

Prices subject to change without notice.

Some Other New Harbinger Self-Help Titles

Multiple Chemical Sensitivity: A Survival Guide, $16.95
Dancing Naked, $14.95
Why Are We Still Fighting, $15.95
From Sabotage to Success, $14.95
Parkinson's Disease and the Art of Moving, $15.95
A Survivor's Guide to Breast Cancer, $13.95
Men, Women, and Prostate Cancer, $15.95
Make Every Session Count: Getting the Most Out of Your Brief Therapy, $10.95
Virtual Addiction, $12.95
After the Breakup, $13.95
Why Can't I Be the Parent I Want to Be?, $12.95
The Secret Message of Shame, $13.95
The OCD Workbook, $18.95
Tapping Your Inner Strength, $13.95
Binge No More, $14.95
When to Forgive, $12.95
Practical Dreaming, $12.95
Healthy Baby, Toxic World, $15.95
Making Hope Happen, $14.95
I'll Take Care of You, $12.95
Survivor Guilt, $14.95
Children Changed by Trauma, $13.95
Understanding Your Child's Sexual Behavior, $12.95
The Self-Esteem Companion, $10.95
The Gay and Lesbian Self-Esteem Book, $13.95
Making the Big Move, $13.95
How to Survive and Thrive in an Empty Nest, $13.95
Living Well with a Hidden Disability, $15.95
Overcoming Repetitive Motion Injuries the Rossiter Way, $15.95
What to Tell the Kids About Your Divorce, $13.95
The Divorce Book, Second Edition, $15.95
Claiming Your Creative Self: True Stories from the Everyday Lives of Women, $15.95
Six Keys to Creating the Life You Desire, $19.95
Taking Control of TMJ, $13.95
What You Need to Know About Alzheimer's, $15.95
Winning Against Relapse: A Workbook of Action Plans for Recurring Health and Emotional Problems, $14.95
Facing 30: Women Talk About Constructing a Real Life and Other Scary Rites of Passage, $12.95
The Worry Control Workbook, $15.95
Wanting What You Have: A Self-Discovery Workbook, $18.95
When Perfect Isn't Good Enough: Strategies for Coping with Perfectionism, $13.95
Earning Your Own Respect: A Handbook of Personal Responsibility, $12.95
High on Stress: A Woman's Guide to Optimizing the Stress in Her Life, $13.95
Infidelity: A Survival Guide, $13.95
Stop Walking on Eggshells, $14.95
Consumer's Guide to Psychiatric Drugs, $16.95
The Fibromyalgia Advocate: Getting the Support You Need to Cope with Fibromyalgia and Myofascial Pain, $18.95
Healing Fear: New Approaches to Overcoming Anxiety, $16.95
Working Anger: Preventing and Resolving Conflict on the Job, $12.95
Sex Smart: How Your Childhood Shaped Your Sexual Life and What to Do About It, $14.95
You Can Free Yourself From Alcohol & Drugs, $13.95
Amongst Ourselves: A Self-Help Guide to Living with Dissociative Identity Disorder, $14.95
Healthy Living with Diabetes, $13.95
Dr. Carl Robinson's Basic Baby Care, $10.95
Better Boundries: Owning and Treasuring Your Life, $13.95
Goodbye Good Girl, $12.95
Fibromyalgia & Chronic Myofascial Pain Syndrome, $19.95
The Depression Workbook: Living With Depression and Manic Depression, $17.95
Self-Esteem, Second Edition, $13.95
Angry All the Time: An Emergency Guide to Anger Control, $12.95
When Anger Hurts, $13.95
Perimenopause, $16.95
The Relaxation & Stress Reduction Workbook, Fourth Edition, $17.95
The Anxiety & Phobia Workbook, Second Edition, $18.95
I Can't Get Over It, A Handbook for Trauma Survivors, Second Edition, $16.95
Messages: The Communication Skills Workbook, Second Edition, $15.95
Thoughts & Feelings, Second Edition, $18.95
Depression: How It Happens, How It's Healed, $14.95
The Deadly Diet, Second Edition, $14.95
The Power of Two, $15.95

Call **toll free, 1-800-748-6273**, or log on to our online bookstore at **www.newharbinger.com** to order. Have your Visa or Mastercard number ready. Or send a check for the titles you want to New Harbinger Publications, Inc., 5674 Shattuck Ave., Oakland, CA 94609. Include $3.80 for the first book and 75¢ for each additional book, to cover shipping and handling. (California residents please include appropriate sales tax.) Allow two to five weeks for delivery.

Prices subject to change without notice.